NO EXCUSES
DETOX

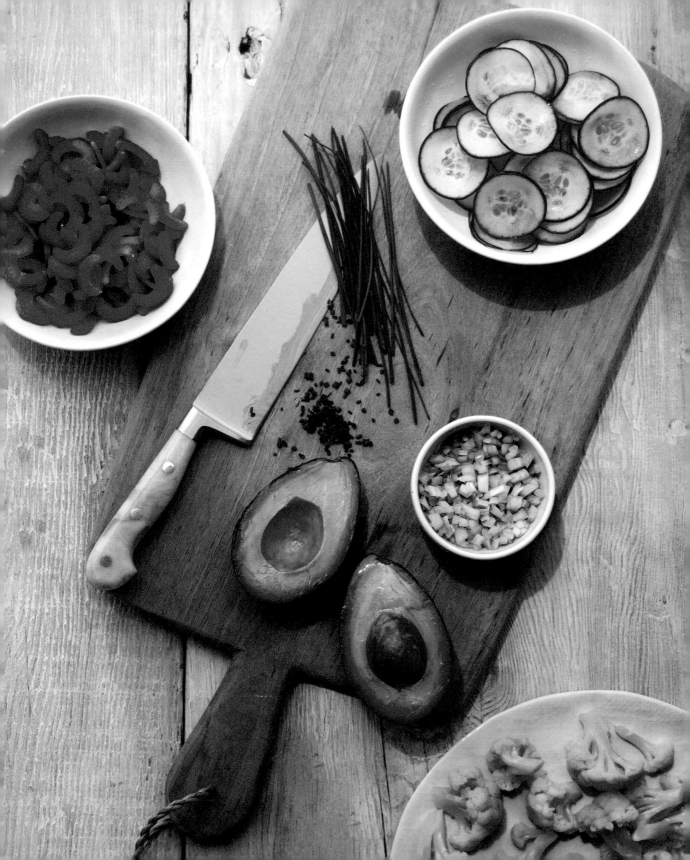

NO EXCUSES
DETOX

100 RECIPES TO HELP YOU
EAT HEALTHY EVERY DAY

MEGAN GILMORE

PHOTOGRAPHS BY ERIN SCOTT

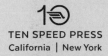

TEN SPEED PRESS
California | New York

TO MY FAMILY, WHO INSPIRES ME EACH DAY TO CREATE HEALTHFUL AND DELICIOUS MEALS, EVEN WHEN I'M FEELING "TOO BUSY."

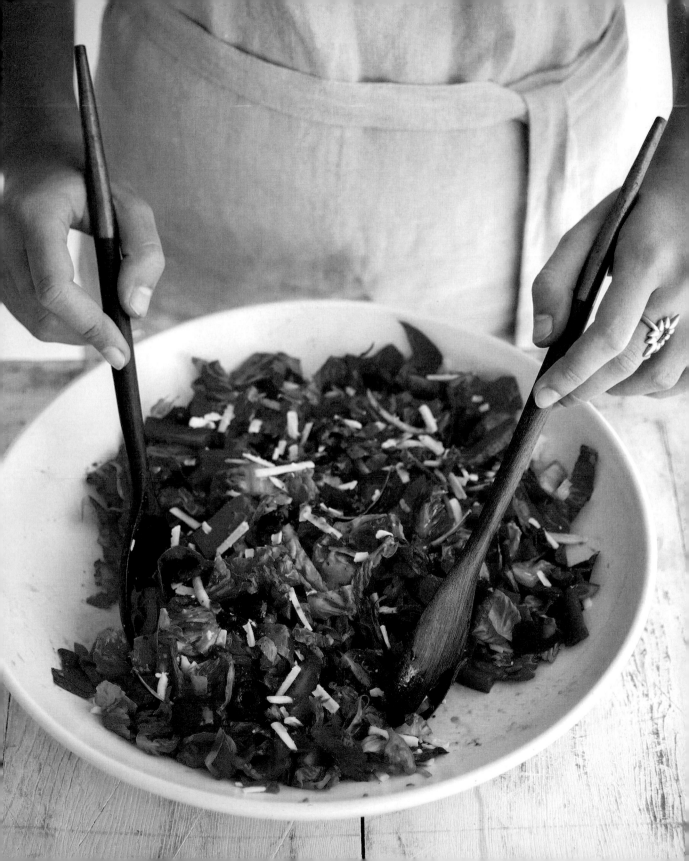

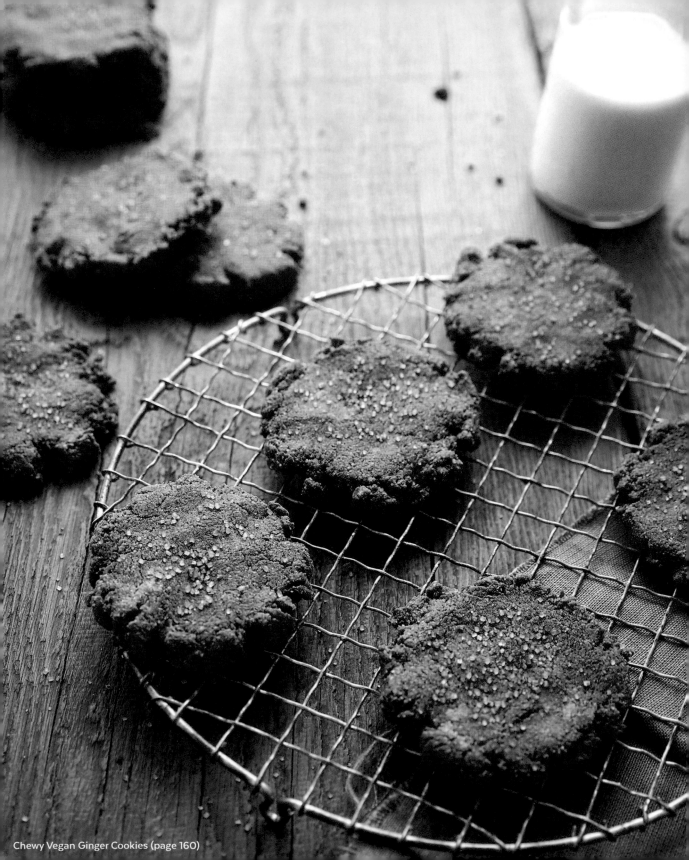

Chewy Vegan Ginger Cookies (page 160)

CONTENTS

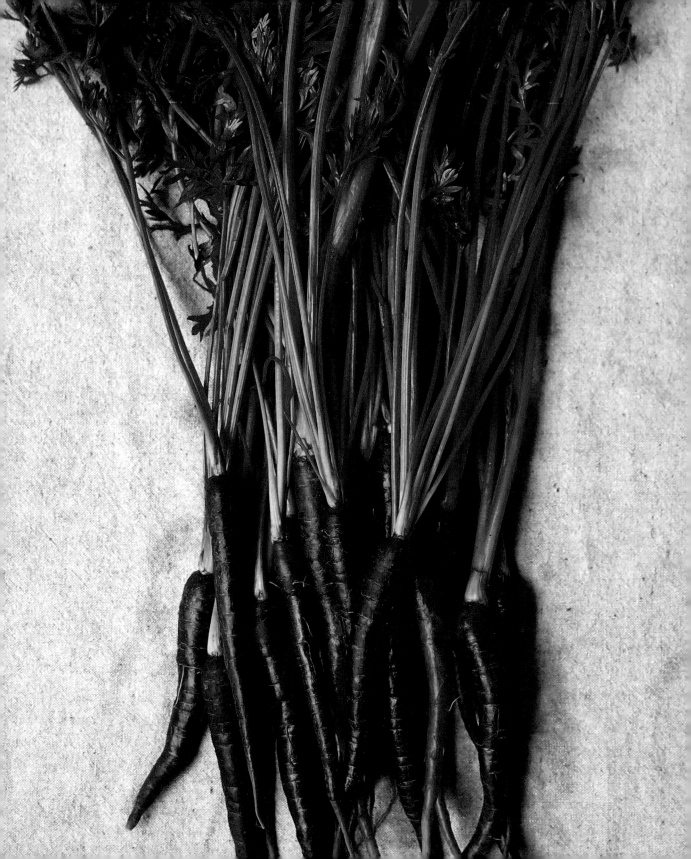

1 NO MORE EXCUSES

In our busy world, it's not always easy to eat healthy. Even though healthful foods are more abundant and more accessible than ever before, everyday triggers such as stress, finances, social events, and an overall lack of time often get in the way when it comes to making good food choices. But not anymore. In this book, I'll share solutions to help you combat those everyday excuses and make healthy eating easier than ever.

HOW WILL THIS HELP YOU DETOX? Not only will you be ridding yourself of the excuses that hold you back but you'll also reduce your exposure to toxins when you make better eating choices. As you may know, we are exposed to a host of environmental toxins on a daily basis, including pollution, mold, phthalates, VOCs (volatile organic compounds), heavy metals, and more. While we can't always control our exposure to these environmental pollutants, what we can control is how much additional work we pile on to our body's natural detoxification system by avoiding foods that contain chemical dyes, preservatives, and toxic packaging.

If you're familiar with my first book, *Everyday Detox*, you know that my approach to detoxing is different from most. Instead of taking drastic measures for thirty days or less, you will enjoy delicious and satisfying meals made from whole foods all year long. When you increase your consumption of organic, fresh foods and reduce your intake of the refined and processed variety, you'll reduce the load placed on your crucial detox organs so they can function at their peak. No gimmicky cleanses required.

In fact, many of those popular short-term cleanses and detox programs may be holding you back because you're avoiding the real task at hand—making lasting lifestyle changes. While juice fasts and other cleanses may have their benefits, it's far more important to learn how to feed yourself well on a regular basis. That's what is so special about this no-excuse approach to detoxing. There's no need to wait for the perfect time to cleanse. You won't need to isolate yourself from social situations or fear

forbidden food temptations because eating this way won't disrupt your daily life. No matter what your schedule or excuse, you can always find a way to eat healthful food in real-life situations. (Of course, whether you always "want to" is another story . . . just don't use it as an excuse.)

The recipes in this book have all been developed with speed, convenience, and cost in mind to make healthy eating as easy as possible. While I do enjoy cooking, I'm also a busy working mom and don't have all day to spend in the kitchen—and I know you don't either. My family members will only eat meals that taste really good (in other words, they can't taste too "healthy"), and, like most families, we also need to stick to a budget. So, rest assured that all of your concerns will be addressed in the following chapters, and that eating real food in real-life situations is totally doable, even with a crazy schedule.

Despite the ease of this approach, I know how tempting it can be to put it off for one more day, so let's tackle your excuses right away. Because let's be honest, most of the things that hold us back are just that—excuses!

While I can't do the work for you, I will do my best to provide realistic solutions to help you make the changes necessary to succeed. In the recipe chapters, we'll tackle the logistical side of things so you can experience firsthand that preparing healthy food can be quick, affordable, and delicious. But first, let's discuss the mental roadblocks that may be keeping you from consistently sticking to your healthy living goals.

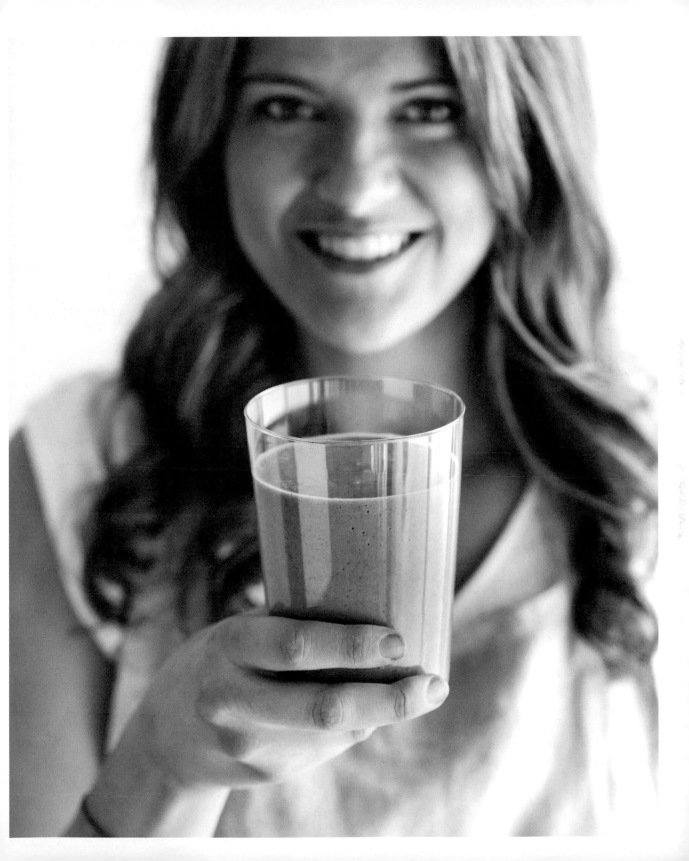

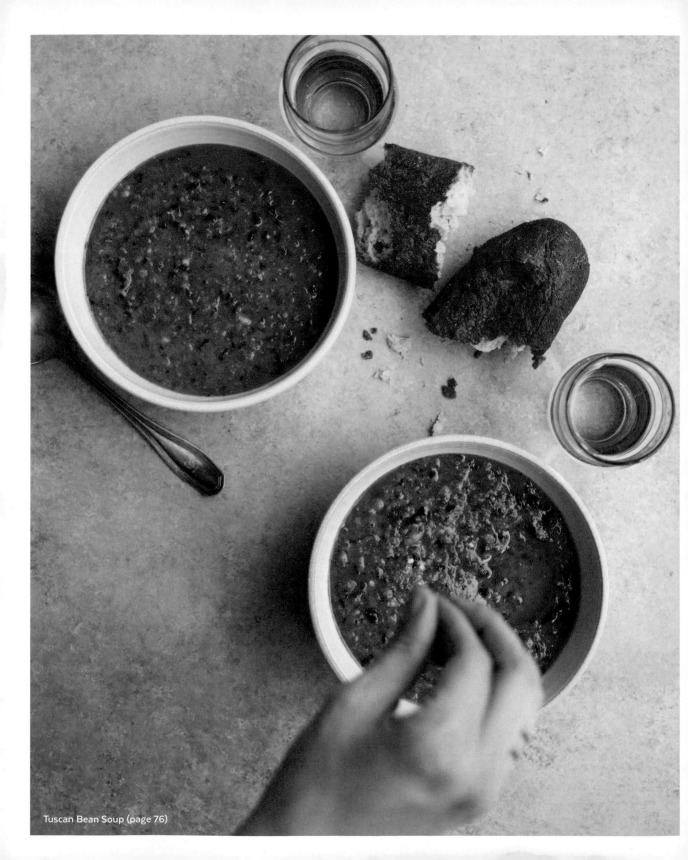

Tuscan Bean Soup (page 76)

THE TOP FIVE MOST COMMON EXCUSES

To get started, let's focus on the top five most common excuses I hear from my readers and nutrition clients when it comes to not eating well on a regular basis. Many of them might sound familiar to you, too.

EXCUSE #1: I DON'T HAVE ENOUGH TIME

Not having enough time is by far the most common excuse out there, and with good reason. As a society, we are busier than ever, and cooking healthful meals from scratch can certainly be more time-consuming than picking up a prepared meal on the way home from work or heating up a frozen pizza. However, I'm guessing that most of you reading this book do have at least thirty minutes to spare if you're willing to make healthy eating a priority. Perhaps you could prep your meals for the week while watching a thirty-minute show on Netflix? That's multitasking at its finest.

Here are a few easy tips to squeeze healthy eating into your busy schedule.

- **Seek out speedy recipes.** Many of the recipes in this book are labeled with a Thirty-Minute Recipe icon to help you locate dishes that are ready from start-to-finish in just, you guessed it, thirty minutes. Other recipes require just fifteen minutes of hands-on preparation so you can be productive doing other things around the house while your meal bakes to perfection in the oven. If you can't find fifteen minutes to spare for yourself each night, you may need to reorganize your priorities a bit to make that possible.

- **Make good use of your freezer.** Have you ever heard the phrase, "Cook once, enjoy twice"? It should be the motto of every busy home cook. Make the most of your hands-on time by preparing double batches of your favorite recipes and freezing the extras for fast and easy future meals. Keep an eye out throughout this book for the Freezer-Friendly label denoting recipes that freeze well.

- **Take advantage of healthful convenience foods.** Most grocery stores now offer a wide variety of prewashed and prechopped packaged vegetables, so if you don't have time to prep your own veggies, they are still incredibly easy to come by. When possible, be sure to look for ingredients, such as tomato paste, that come packaged in glass jars. This will help you avoid any chemicals potentially found in metal can linings. Also, be sure to check out your grocer's freezer section. Many now offer cooked grains frozen into individual serving sizes, sliced stir-fry vegetables, and precooked meats, so a healthier freezer meal is only minutes away when you're crunched for time.

The next time you think you're "too busy" to eat well, what you're really saying is that healthy eating isn't a priority for you at that moment. If you think about it, it would probably take you at least twenty minutes to get in the car and return home with food from a drive-thru window, so there's no reason why you can't use that time more wisely to whip up a healthy and satisfying dinner that won't weigh you down. With all of the healthy and convenient options available, not having enough time is no longer a good excuse to sacrifice eating well.

EXCUSE #2: IT'S TOO EXPENSIVE

It's true that fresh organic produce is more expensive than the conventionally grown variety and that pasture-raised animal products are more expensive than factory-farmed animal products. However, that doesn't mean that healthy eating has to break the bank.

In the recipe chapters, I share plenty of budget-friendly meal ideas (along with the price per serving, so you can budget accordingly), so don't be surprised if your grocery bill goes down simply by preparing more whole-food meals at home. Many packaged foods, such as potato chips, sodas, and cookies—especially those with a brand name or a "healthy" marketing label—are more expensive than simply choosing whole foods in the first place.

Here are a few more ways you can save money while eating well.

- **Stick to a meal plan.** I've included three complete weeks of meal plans and shopping lists (starting on page 20) to help you stay on track and on budget. When you shop for only the items you need each week, you'll avoid making expensive impulse purchases, and you won't need to dine out when you find yourself hungry and unprepared. Preparation is key, so take twenty minutes out of your weekend to plan your meals for the week along with a corresponding grocery list.

- **Eat fewer animal products.** Animal products, including meat, fish, dairy, and eggs, tend to be the priciest items in a shopping cart, so by reducing your weekly consumption you can easily shave dollars off your grocery bill while also potentially increasing your life span.[1] If your family relies heavily on meat-centered dishes, try serving a little less meat at each

meal and then make up the difference by adding extra veggies to your plates. Or, simply aim to eat "meatless" one day a week and try a new vegetarian meal instead. You'll save money while expanding your palate.

- **Keep it simple.** In my experience, healthful eating is often the most expensive when people are first starting out because they want to dive in headfirst, trying exotic ingredients and packaged convenience foods that are reminiscent of their old favorites. In many cases, these packaged foods aren't much healthier than their processed counterparts, and you certainly don't need a bunch of exotic ingredients to make truly delicious, healthy food. Instead, shop for simple whole foods, such as fresh produce, raw nuts and seeds, and bulk grains, and then use them to make your own salad dressings, dips, snack bars, and puddings for healthier and cheaper alternatives to pricey packaged snacks. This book is loaded with easy recipes for you to do just that.

- **Shop seasonally.** You've probably heard that it's better to eat seasonally and locally, and one of the best benefits of this practice is that it saves you money. When produce is in season, its supply is at its peak—making it easier and cheaper for farmers to distribute to your local store. Those savings get passed on to you, and, as added perks, your food tastes better and is more nutritious. When your favorite produce isn't in season, you can save money by buying it frozen, which is almost always cheaper than fresh.

- **Know the Dirty Dozen.** If you can't afford to buy organic produce all the time, but you want to reduce your exposure to pesticides, familiarize yourself with the "Dirty Dozen" list produced by the Environmental Working Group, a nonprofit environmental research organization. Each year they create this free resource to let consumers know the top twelve fruits and vegetables that are most heavily sprayed with pesticides. They also share a "Clean 15" list, which includes the fifteen items that are least exposed to pesticides. Using these lists as your guide, you can save money by buying organic only when shopping for highly sprayed produce. Visit www.ewg.org to print your own copy. If you don't have the Dirty Dozen list on hand when shopping for produce, a good way to determine if choosing organic is worth the extra money is to think about how you will eat it. If you're going to eat the skin, such as an apple or a bell pepper, buy organic. If you need to peel the fruit or vegetable, such as a squash or an avocado, conventional produce is just fine, since you'll be discarding the peel and a majority of the pesticide residue along with it.

When you start to make healthful eating a priority, you will most likely cut back on some other expensive habits, such as dining out often, buying triple-shot skinny-mocha lattes with whipped cream, eating greasy popcorn at the movie theater, or sipping overpriced cocktails. Improving your health now will likely mean fewer costly doctor visits for you in the future, too. Consider that even more reason to banish this "too expensive" excuse for good.

EXCUSE #3: MY FAMILY IS TOO PICKY

Even if you're the only person in your home who wants to eat healthier, you shouldn't have to become a short-order cook. It may take time for everyone in your household to make the transition, but gradually introducing higher-quality foods and trying a new recipe each week is a great way to help your family establish healthier eating habits while expanding their palates. Make it a priority!

Try some of these easy ways to get started. The more consistent you are, the faster you'll see positive results!

- **Sneak in some green.** Add a handful of fresh baby spinach to your family's favorite fruit smoothie. You'll benefit from the added nutrients, and you won't be able to taste the greens at all. If you or your family members are leery of green drinks, include frozen blueberries or raw cacao powder to completely mask the color. (Be sure to try the Frosty Chocolate Shake on page 30.)

- **Bulk up your plate with veggies.** Replace half of your pasta with zucchini "noodles" (try the Rainbow Lo Mein on page 147) or steamed vegetables to boost the fiber and nutrients in your meal, while still indulging in a hearty pasta dish. Eventually, you might be surprised that you prefer a higher ratio of vegetables to pasta on your plate. The same technique may also be used with rice dishes—replace half of the white or brown rice with cauliflower "rice" for an easy vegetable boost that doesn't significantly change the overall taste or texture of your family's favorite meals.

- **Keep healthful snacks in sight.** Arrange fresh fruit on the counter and sliced veggies with dip in your refrigerator as easy-to-grab snack options. Keep your fridge filled with healthy foods at eye level so they are the first option you see when you open the door. I do this for my toddler by keeping a batch of prepared smoothies, applesauce pouches, and sliced fruit in our fridge door at his eye level so he can "independently" choose a healthy snack. It's empowering to give everyone the choice.

- **Make new and "kid-friendly" recipes.** I have several kid-friendly options labeled throughout this book—and they're adult-approved, too. Butternut Mac 'n' Cheese (page 122) is a creamy and tasty alternative to the boxed neon-orange kind and packs some veggies into each bite. It's also hard to resist a serving of delicious Philly Cheesesteak-Stuffed Spaghetti Squash (page 121), my Chocolate Sweet Potato Buttercream (page 168) with a sneaky vegetable base, or Creamy "Peanut" Dressing (see page 70)—it always has everyone reaching for more veggies to dip into it. Try new recipes often because you never know what new dish your family might enjoy until you try it.

- **Keep meals flexible.** I refuse to be a short-order cook, but I have no problem modifying a dish I'm already making to accommodate my family members. For example, my husband prefers to eat meat more often than I do, so I will add a precooked chicken breast to his portion to help him feel satisfied, while keeping my portion vegetarian. Or if he feels the need for more bulk when I'm serving a dish made with cauliflower rice, I'll use an individual portion of frozen cooked rice from our freezer to add to his plate. It's not much extra work on my part, and he's still getting a mostly vegetable-centric meal without feeling overwhelmed by drastic diet changes. There's no need to prepare an entirely different meal.

EXCUSE #4: I'M ALWAYS ON THE GO

If you have to travel often for work, feel as if you're always in your car, or simply aren't around your kitchen much, you can still eat well on the go—as long as you make it a priority. Sticking to your healthy eating goals is more important than ever when you're on the go because your immune system is closely tied to your gut health. When you eat nutrient-rich foods, you'll give your immune system a much-needed boost and help reduce your chances of catching a cold, even if you're exposed to more germs than usual in a crowded dance studio, child's soccer game, or busy airport. (Be sure to get plenty of sleep, too.)

Here are a few on-the-go tips to help you stay well and on track.

- **Choose healthful portable snacks.** Fresh fruit is nature's ultimate "fast food" since it's already packed for you in an easily portable skin. Apples, bananas, pears, and oranges are all widely available—even at gas stations and coffee chains—and can be stored at room temperature for days. There's no reason why you can't pack several pieces in your suitcase, purse, or car to enjoy a nutrient-rich snack anytime. (If you're worried about the sugar naturally found in fruit, be sure to see my note on page 33.) Raw nuts, seeds, and dried fruits are also easy portable options, and you can usually find them available in airport kiosks and vending machines for a quick and easy snack.

- **Make your own snacks.** My Date Energy Bites (page 111) and Nut-Free Chewy Granola Bars (page 112) are a breeze to prepare and pack well on the go. They also happen to taste like dessert, so you won't feel deprived while you're out. If you're craving something salty, try the Easy Party Mix (page 103) for a more satiating alternative to chips.

- **Dine out wisely.** It's likely that you'll need to dine out while traveling or going to a post-game celebration, but luckily for you, there are still plenty of restaurants and fast-food chains that offer healthier choices.

Common real-food options include steamed or grilled veggies, leafy green salads, broth-based vegetable or lentil soups, black beans, guacamole, salsa, plain baked potatoes, vegetable omelets, and more. If you don't see what you want on the menu, don't be afraid to ask. Many places are happy to accommodate your needs if you ask them nicely enough.

> **Traveling for a Vacation?**
>
> Now that's a different story. I think it's reasonable to assume that most of us vacation only once or twice a year, and in that case, I encourage you to indulge in the local fare and create once-in-a-lifetime memories with your friends and loved ones without worrying about your diet. There's no need to be a perfectionist while on vacation. It's what you do consistently in the long run that counts.

If you find yourself traveling often or dining out several times a week, those daily indulgences can quickly start to take their toll on your energy levels and overall quality of life. However, when you start to take care of yourself by using the previous tips, the better you'll feel and the more you'll want to stick to your healthy eating plan. Start building up your momentum now because it does get easier the more you practice.

EXCUSE #5: I CAN'T CONTROL MY CRAVINGS

Whether you're on a diet or not, it's totally natural to crave a sweet treat or salty snack every now and then. However, if your cravings feel out of control or start to occur more frequently, there could be a valid reason why.

The following issues might help you get to the bottom of your cravings.

- **You're not eating enough.** Many dieters are chronically undernourished after attempting a calorie-restricted regimen because they're simply not eating enough food to get the nutrients they need in the first place. Calorie counting is a flawed approach because it doesn't take the nutrient density of your food into account, and studies have shown that exposure to toxins can prompt weight gain regardless of calorie intake or exercise.[2] Instead of counting calories, focus on nutrient-rich whole foods and eat until you feel satisfied, without worrying about the numbers. You might be surprised to feel your cravings vanish as you enjoy plenty of nourishing foods, and you may find that your taste for sweet and salty foods will diminish as your taste buds adapt, without stressing about portion control.

- **Your food choices are too restrictive.** If you suffer from an all-or-nothing mentality, you might be creating unnecessary cravings by labeling certain foods as "forbidden," even when you're only aiming to adopt a whole-foods diet. By embarking on a super-strict eating regimen, you give certain foods more attention than they deserve simply by proclaiming them off-limits. Instead of taking drastic measures, try making small changes on a daily basis, such as starting your day with a green smoothie, replacing your usual crunchy vending-machine snack with a handful of raw almonds, or indulging in a piece of 5-Minute Freezer Fudge (page 164) instead of a candy bar. Though it might not sound as exciting as committing to a strict cleanse, making these small changes, even with room for some of your favorite treats, will leave you with permanent results that will have everyone wanting to know what "cleanse" you're doing. Even better, you won't ever have to worry about rebounding back into old habits or into a larger clothing size, because practicing manageable new habits on a regular basis is what makes them stick for good.

- **You have food allergies or sensitivities.** Did you know that it's not uncommon to crave foods that you are allergic or intolerant to? It's one of nature's cruel jokes. Food allergies cause stress to the body, and then the body releases endorphins to help make you feel better. The result is that you associate the food you're allergic to with "feeling good," and that may actually make you crave it more. If you suspect that one of your cravings might be related to a food intolerance or allergy, particularly one of the common allergens like wheat or dairy, try an elimination diet to see how your body reacts without it. You may not know how good you can feel until you give it a try.

ONE MORE THING THAT SEEMS TO STALL PEOPLE'S PROGRESS?

- **They don't know where to start.** There's so much conflicting nutritional information out there that it's easy to stall because you don't know which approach to healthful eating is best. The Paleo Diet? A vegan diet? Our society suffers from information overload, and the flood of conflicting studies and theories is enough to make your head spin. Don't use this as another "excuse" to procrastinate changing your habits. Instead, stick to what most experts agree to be true: eat whole foods—with an emphasis on plants—as much as possible. It's hard to go wrong with that approach!

What Is an Elimination Diet?

An elimination diet is one of the most noninvasive ways to determine if you are sensitive to a certain ingredient or food category. Remove common allergens such as gluten, peanuts, dairy, and soy; preservatives such as nitrates and MSG; and any other possible suspects from your diet. For the most accurate results, it's crucial that you stick to this for a minimum of six weeks to make sure your body has had the chance to remove any remaining traces of these ingredients—no cheating! After the six weeks, you'll gradually add each

ingredient back into your diet one week at a time to see if that certain food has an impact on how you feel. After you've reintroduced each ingredient, you can determine for yourself which foods make you feel best. Of course, even if you get to the root of your cravings, it doesn't mean you'll never find yourself wanting a sweet treat or salty snack ever again. Every food choice you make is just that—a choice—and it's what you choose to do regularly that counts. Don't beat yourself up over a treat every now and then and don't let this excuse get in the way of your goals.

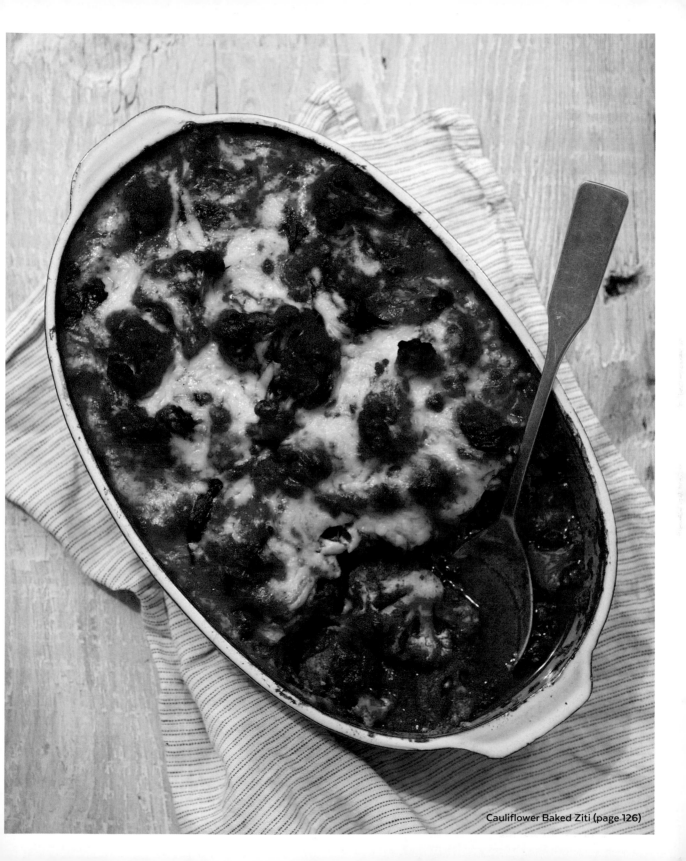

Cauliflower Baked Ziti (page 126)

HOW TO USE THIS BOOK

All of the recipes in this book are naturally gluten-free and vegetarian, but many of them also are written to accommodate omnivores and vegans alike. Be sure to check the bottom of each recipe for substitution notes and meat-friendly options to suit your needs. You can also find nutrition information for each recipe at the end of this book, starting on page 194.

In an effort to make this book as user-friendly (and as excuse-proof) as possible, you'll find the estimated price per serving listed on each recipe to help you stick to your budget, and I've also labeled all of the recipes with common allergy concerns using the following icons:

DF	DAIRY-FREE	**SF**	SOY-FREE
EF	EGG-FREE	**NS**	NO SUGAR
GF	GLUTEN-FREE	**V**	VEGAN
NF	NUT-FREE		

The following criteria are also clearly labeled where appropriate to help make meal planning easier:

30-MINUTE RECIPE

15-MINUTE PREP

KID-FRIENDLY

FREEZER-FRIENDLY

SLOW/PRESSURE COOKER OPTION

SUBSTITUTIONS

Dairy Products

In these recipes, I rely on goat- and sheep-milk products, since they are much easier to digest than cow's milk (see the note on page 50). However, I know these products can sometimes be difficult to locate or don't appeal to everyone's taste buds, so feel free to use cow's dairy in their place if you prefer. Parmesan cheese makes an excellent alternative to Pecorino Romano, and soft feta cheese can be used to replace the soft goat cheese in most recipes.

Gluten-Free Baking

It's best not to make any substitutions regarding gluten-free flour, since coconut flour, almond flour, and oat flour all work significantly differently and could lead to disastrous results if you attempt to replace them. I would hate for you to waste your ingredients. If a recipe calls for a liquid sweetener, like maple syrup, or a granulated sweetener, like coconut sugar, don't be tempted to swap them or use a zero-calorie sweetener without expecting a significantly different, and possibly terrible, outcome. I've made every effort to include as many egg-free recipes in this book as possible, so it's safe to assume that when a recipe calls for eggs, like my Cashew Butter Spice Muffins (page 43), it will not work nearly as well with an egg substitute. Experiment at your own risk!

Cooking Oils

I use coconut oil in many of my recipes because it's such a stable cooking oil, but feel free to use olive oil when cooking, if you prefer (see note on page 115). Do not replace the coconut oil with olive oil in any

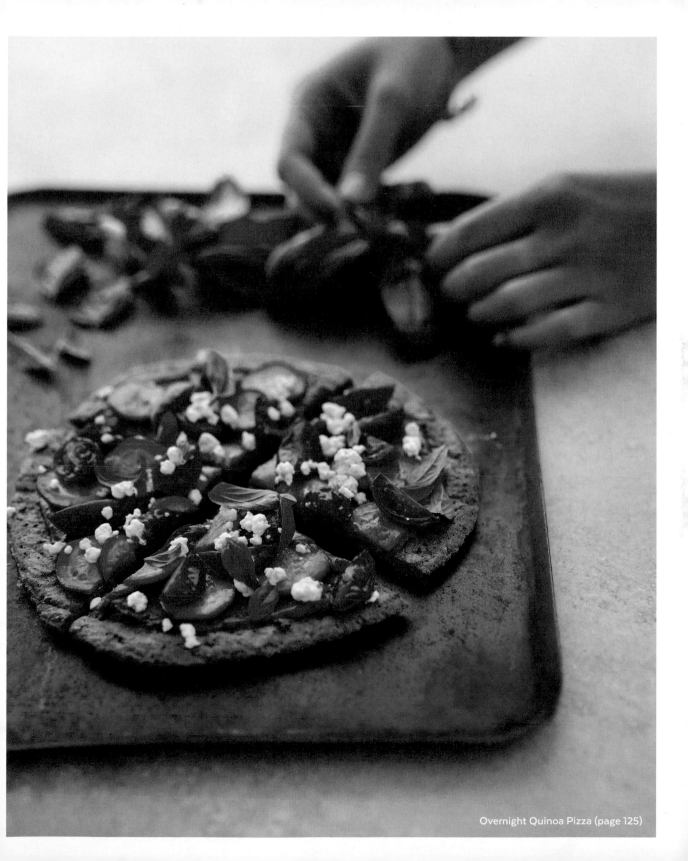

Overnight Quinoa Pizza (page 125)

no-bake recipe or freezer recipe, as the saturated fat found in coconut oil is necessary for the texture in those cases. The best substitute for coconut oil in no-bake recipes is real butter, as it is also solid at room temperature.

Cacao versus Cocoa Powder

When it comes to chocolate recipes, I always call for raw cacao powder in recipes that won't be heated, to maximize the nutritional benefits found in this unprocessed ingredient, but flavor-wise I find raw cacao powder and cocoa powder to be interchangeable. In recipes that will be heated, such as the Vegan Chocolate Cake on page 166, I prefer to use the more affordable cocoa powder as it will be exposed to high temperatures, which can compromise certain nutrients.

Soy

If you can't tolerate soy, you may use coconut aminos as a soy-free replacement for tamari in any recipe. Keep in mind that coconut aminos have a milder flavor than the gluten-free soy sauce, so you'll need to season the dish with extra salt to compensate. (See Resources at the back of the book for brand recommendations.)

Nut-Free

To make a recipe nut-free, you may use Sunflower Butter (page 187) in place of most nut butters, but keep in mind that sunflower seeds are more bitter in flavor, so you'll need to adjust the recipe to taste when making that substitution. Also, sunflower seeds have a unique (but safe) reaction with baking soda that turns baked goods green, so be prepared for that!

Quickly Cook Sweet Potatoes

To prepare sweet potatoes quickly in an electric pressure cooker, stab each potato several times with a fork to help them vent. Add 1 cup water to cover the bottom of the pressure cooker bowl and arrange the potatoes in a metal steamer basket, or use the metal insert that comes with the Instant Pot. Secure the lid, making sure the vent is closed, and cook on high pressure for 10 minutes, or until tender. Allow the pressure to release naturally before carefully removing the lid. To bake your potatoes, stab each potato several times with a fork to help them vent, rub with a bit of coconut oil, and place them on a baking sheet. Bake in a 400°F oven until tender, 45 to 60 minutes, depending on size. The potatoes are done when they are easily pierced with a fork.

Quickly Cook Spaghetti Squash

In an electric pressure cooker, add 1 cup water to cover the bottom of the pot. Cut the squash in half and scoop out the seeds, then place the halves in a metal steamer basket. Secure the lid, making sure the vent is closed, and cook on high pressure for 10 minutes, or until the shell of the squash is easily pierced with a fork. Allow the pressure to release naturally before removing the lid. If you don't have a pressure cooker, you can bake the squash up to 4 days in advance. Place the cut and seeded squash halves cut-side down on a baking sheet and bake in a 400°F oven until the shell is easily pierced with a fork, about 45 minutes. A good sign that the halves are done is that a large brown spot will develop on the outside shell.

FREEZER OR SLOW/PRESSURE COOKER METHOD

Many of the recipes in this book have been tested as freezer meals, but some work better than others, which is why I've denoted when a recipe is freezer-friendly or not. Regardless of the recipe, the process is pretty similar across the board so I've outlined the general steps here for easy reference. Keep in mind that if you are preparing a meal to impress guests or picky eaters, I recommend making the recipe fresh from scratch, as reheated vegetarian freezer meals will always be slightly more muted in flavor and mushier in texture. However, they are a real time-saver on busy weeknights!

For best results and even cooking, thaw the frozen meal in the fridge overnight before reheating.

To freeze: For best results, sauté the aromatic ingredients such as onions, celery, and garlic, along with any seasonings like curry powder. (This is usually found in step 1 or 2 of most recipes.) Transfer the cooked aromatics to a freezer safe 1-gallon container and add in the rest of the ingredients, other than large amounts of liquid, such as canned coconut milk or water. Freeze in an airtight container for up to 6 months, and for even cooking be sure to thaw the frozen meal in the fridge overnight before reheating.

To reheat in a slow/pressure cooker: Dump the thawed contents into the cooker bowl and add any remaining liquid called for in the recipe. In a slow cooker, cook on high temperature for 3 hours or low for 6 hours. In a pressure cooker, cook on high pressure for 10 minutes with the lid securely sealed, and allow the pressure to release naturally before carefully removing the lid. Once the food is heated through, stir in any remaining ingredients and adjust the seasoning to taste before serving.

To reheat on the stove top: Dump the thawed contents into a large Dutch oven placed over medium heat and add any remaining liquid called for. Stir until the dish is heated through, then adjust the seasonings to taste and serve warm. In the case of a soup, or a recipe with lentils, bring the liquid to a boil to incorporate the seasonings and ensure every ingredient is tender before serving.

To cook from scratch in a slow cooker or pressure cooker:
For best results and to bring out a rich flavor, sauté aromatic ingredients such as onions, celery, and garlic, and seasonings like curry powder before placing everything into the pot. (This is usually found in step 1 or 2 of most recipes.) If you have an electric pressure cooker, such as an Instant Pot, you can sauté directly in the pressure cooker bowl without dirtying an extra pan.

Once the aromatics are tender, add in the remaining ingredients called for, except for those that are instructed to be stirred in at the end, such as nondairy milk or lemon juice. Securely seal the lid according to the manufacturer's instructions. Cook vegetarian meals (including those with red lentils) for 8 minutes on high pressure. Cook meals with raw chopped meat for 10 minutes on high pressure. Allow the pressure to release naturally, then carefully remove the lid. Adjust any seasonings to taste and serve warm.

FOOD-COMBINING CHEAT SHEET

For those of you already familiar with my website, detoxinista.com, you know that I strategically develop most of my recipes with optimum digestion in mind, using a practice called food combining. Put simply, food combining is a method of mindfully eating where you keep certain food groups separate to help your digestion run more smoothly. Studies have shown that humans have a tendency to overeat when they are offered a wide variety of foods during a meal.[3] So, by minimizing the variety of foods on your plate at each meal, you will naturally eat less, without counting calories or worrying about portion sizes. This is perhaps why so many people who start practicing food combining tend to reach their ideal weight, even without counting calories.

You can read about food combining in more detail in my first book, *Everyday Detox*, but if you want to start following along right away, I've included a quick cheat sheet on the facing page.

For the purposes of this book, food combining is optional because I know it can seem complicated or overwhelming at first, and I don't want you to use that as another "excuse" to put off healthful eating for another day. If you follow the meal plans in this book, along with the recipes, the food-combining aspect has already been done for you—so it's a no-brainer! Each recipe is clearly labeled for how it combines. However, if you want to add meat, cheese, nuts, or a handful of fruit to any of these healthy recipes, that's fine, too. If you ask me, it's far more important that you truly enjoy the experience of every meal you eat, so that you create an overall positive association with healthy eating. If a mis-combined dish keeps you consistently eating higher-quality whole foods, that's still a step in the right direction.

In fact, I've labeled a small selection of the recipes in this book as a "Special Treat" because they don't follow strict food-combining rules. These recipes are still an upgrade from traditional favorites because they use whole-food ingredients, but they are not intended to be eaten on an everyday basis.

AT EACH MEAL CHOOSE TO EAT FROM ONE OF THE FOLLOWING FOUR CATEGORIES:

STARCHES

Acorn Squash · Amaranth · Barley · Beans · Buckwheat · Butternut Squash · Cereals · Cooked Corn · Kabocha Squash · Lentils · Millet Oats · Pasta · Quinoa · Rice · Rye · Spelt · Sweet Potatoes · Wheat White Potatoes · Yams · Young Thai Coconut Meat

ANIMAL PROTEIN

Cheese · Eggs · Fish
Ice Cream · Milk · Pork
Poultry · Red Meat · Yogurt

FRESH FRUIT

Apples · Avocados
Bananas · Berries
Grapefruit · Grapes · Kiwi
Mango · Melons · Nectarines
Oranges · Papaya · Peaches
Pears · Pineapple

NUTS / SEEDS / DRIED FRUIT

Almonds · Brazil Nuts · Cashews · Chia Seeds
Coconut (dried and mature) · Dried Fruit · Flax Seeds · Hazelnuts
Hemp Seeds · Macadamia Nuts · Pecans · Sesame Seeds
Sunflower Seeds · Walnuts

Any of these categories may be combined with "neutral" leafy greens and raw or cooked nonstarchy vegetables to complete your meal. As an easy reference, most vegetables that you can enjoy raw, such as broccoli, carrots, lettuce, zucchini, and more, can be considered neutral. A small condiment also won't have a huge impact on your digestion, so feel free to add a pat of butter to your baked potato or a splash of almond milk to your porridge any time.

Wait three to four hours before switching categories, but feel free to snack on neutral vegetables at any time of the day.

BUT, THERE ARE EXCEPTIONS TO THE RULE:

- Bananas usually digest well with nuts, seeds, and dried fruit.

- Avocados can digest well with fresh fruit, dried fruit, or starches.

- Spaghetti squash is hydrating enough to be considered neutral.

- Peanuts and soy nuts are not recommended due to their potential exposure to pesticides and mold.

TIME-SAVING TIPS

USE A PRESSURE COOKER

An electric pressure cooker is similar to a slow cooker but way faster. Grains, potatoes, and meats cook in just 10 to 12 minutes in a pressure cooker, and nonstarchy vegetables are steamed in just 3 minutes—even faster than using your stove top. Use a pressure cooker to your advantage by preparing large batches of grains and potatoes to store for easy meals during the week, or prepare a last-minute soup or stew (such as the Mock Mulligatawny Stew on page 81) in just 15 minutes on a busy night.

PREP-AS-YOU-GO

You'll notice that many recipes require that you sauté an onion for 8 to 10 minutes before moving on to the next step, so use that time to chop the rest of the veggies needed for the recipe. There's no need to do it all ahead of time. Using this method, you need to chop only an onion before diving into a recipe, which can save you valuable time and help you get dinner on the table as quickly as possible.

BAKE SEVERAL ITEMS AT ONCE

Unless you use the previous pressure cooker tip, preparing a baked sweet potato or spaghetti squash usually takes 45 to 60 minutes of baking time. Rather than baking them individually as needed for a recipe, bake them together all at once, so you can knock out both in only an hour, when you would be at home anyway. I like to do this on the weekend, so I have precooked squash and potatoes ready to go in the refrigerator for a faster weeknight meal. When you have these items on hand, the Spinach & Artichoke "Pasta" Bake (page 120), Philly Cheesesteak-Stuffed Spaghetti Squash (page 121), and Sloppy Joe–Stuffed Sweet Potatoes (page 118) come together in no time.

REPEAT YOUR MEALS

If you're pressed for time, make the most of it by preparing a double batch of any meal you're cooking. Then just reheat the leftovers for an even faster meal in the future. The same goes for salad dressings, dips, and snacks, too. The more you can make all at once, the less work you will have to do for the rest of the week—as long as you don't mind eating the same salad dressing or snacks all week long. Stock your freezer with options like Overnight Quinoa Pizza crusts (see page 125), prepared Cauliflower & Leek Soup (page 79), and the filling for Enchilada-Stuffed Zucchini Boats (see page 138) for a quick meal any time, and make a double batch of Creamy Herb Dressing (page 56) to use over your salads and as a veggie dip for snacks.

FREEZE INDIVIDUAL PORTIONS

You'll have no excuse not to eat well when you have single-serving portions waiting for you in your freezer. Freeze 1-cup portions of cooked grains and beans and pair with frozen sliced vegetables for a quick stir-fry, and freeze your favorite curry, pesto, pizza, and pasta sauces into ice-cube trays for easy portioning and reheating. (Thaw four or five cubes per serving.) You can even prepare your smoothies for the week by measuring out the ingredients into individual containers. When you are running late in the morning, all you'll need to do is dump one of them into the blender with water for a quick and healthy breakfast.

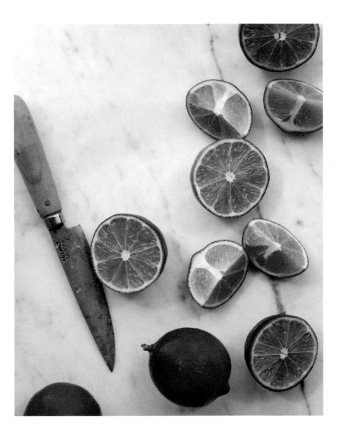

KEEP A SALAD BAR IN YOUR FRIDGE

Chop several heads of lettuce and vegetable toppings at once to store in individual glass containers in your refrigerator, and whip up a large batch of salad dressing in your blender to keep on hand for the week. You'll have an affordable salad bar at your fingertips, making you more likely to eat a salad during the week, even when you're feeling "too busy."

Now, let's tackle your meal plans for the week ahead.

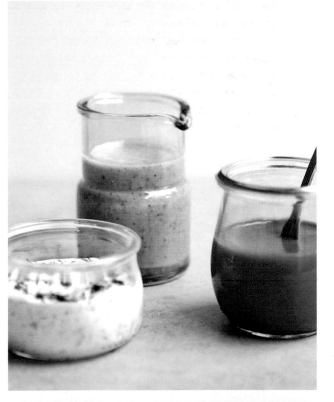

NO-EXCUSES
MEAL PLANS

When it comes to making healthful eating easy, preparation is half of the battle—so I've prepared the following meal plans to help you get started right away. I've included something here for everyone, whether you're a beginner just looking for a variety of easy and delicious meals, you need to stick to a strict budget, or you need to have your meals ready as fast as possible. The more often you practice preparing your own meals, the easier it will get, so let's dive in.

All of the meal plans are accompanied by a corresponding shopping list, but I've also included a general pantry list to the right to make sure you have the basics covered first. You'll notice that I use many of the same ingredients over and over, so as long as you have these essentials on hand, you'll be able to make a wide variety of delicious dishes.

PANTRY SHOPPING LIST

PANTRY STAPLES

Extra-virgin olive oil

Coconut oil

Sesame seed oil (store in refrigerator after opening)

Raw apple cider vinegar

Balsamic vinegar

Honey (clover and raw)

Maple syrup (store in refrigerator after opening)

Dijon mustard (store in refrigerator after opening)

Blackstrap molasses

Tamari (gluten-free soy sauce—store in refrigerator after opening)

Sriracha (store in refrigerator after opening)

Toasted sesame oil

Raw tahini

Raw almond butter

Raw cashew butter

Sunflower seed butter (no sugar added)

Gluten-free rolled oats

Gluten-free oat flour (or just grind your own rolled oats)

Raw cacao powder

Baking soda

Vanilla extract

Ground chia seeds

Ground flax seeds

Hemp hearts

Nutritional yeast (not to be confused with brewer's yeast)

DRIED SPICES

Ground cinnamon

Ground cumin

Ground ginger

Ground nutmeg

Garlic powder

Onion powder

Chili powder

Dried oregano

Dried chives

Dried dill

Paprika

Cayenne pepper

Crushed red pepper flakes

Fine sea salt

Black pepper

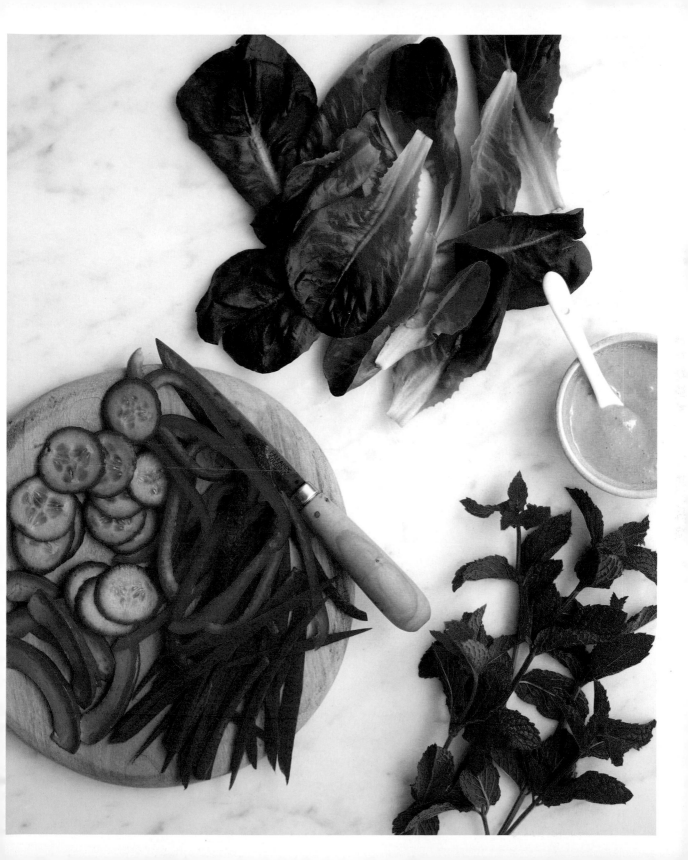

BEGINNER FIVE-DAY MEAL PLAN

This meal plan is for anyone looking for easy and delicious options to help you get started. Be sure to check out my time-saving tips on page 18 and use the Make It Ahead Options to make this week as efficient as possible. Keep in mind that most of the recipes in this book serve four people, with the exception of the smoothies and skillet meals. Be sure to adjust your shopping list as needed to accommodate the number of people in your household. If you're only cooking for one, you might want to make fewer of the meals suggested during the week so you can take full advantage of leftovers!

MAKE IT AHEAD OPTIONS

Creamy "Peanut" Dressing · Date Energy Bites · Freezer Oat Waffles
Mediterranean Quinoa Salad · Nut-Free Gingerbread Granola
Speedy Black Bean Burgers · Zucchini Hummus

MONDAY

Breakfast: Nut-Free Gingerbread Granola (page 38) with nondairy milk

Snack (optional): A ripe banana

Lunch: Crunchy Thai Salad with Creamy "Peanut" Dressing (page 70)

Snack (optional): Sliced veggies served with leftover Creamy "Peanut" Dressing

Dinner: Sloppy Joe–Stuffed Sweet Potatoes (page 118) served with side salad

TUESDAY

Breakfast: Orange-Mango Creamsicle Smoothie (page 34)

Snack (optional): A piece of fruit

Lunch: Mediterranean Quinoa Salad (page 66)

Snack (optional): Baked Parsnip Chips (page 114)

Dinner: Speedy Black Bean Burgers (page 130) with side salad

WEDNESDAY

Breakfast: Broccoli Cheddar Egg Muffins (page 44)

Snack (optional): Sliced veggies

Lunch: Chickpea & Avocado "Egg" Salad (page 61) on gluten-free bread

Snack (optional): Sliced veggies with Zucchini Hummus (page 107)

Dinner: Spinach & Artichoke "Pasta" Bake (page 120) with side salad

THURSDAY

Breakfast: Freezer Oat Waffles (page 49)

Snack (optional): A ripe banana

Lunch: Chopped Salad with Creamy Feta Dressing (page 58)

Snack (optional): Cucumber slices topped with sliced goat cheddar

Dinner: "Cheesy" Broccoli Quinoa Casserole (page 140) with side salad

FRIDAY

Breakfast: Frosty Chocolate Shake (page 30)

Snack (optional): One Date Energy Bite (page 111)

Lunch: Southwest Lettuce Wraps with Sweet Cilantro Dressing (page 104)

Snack (optional): Carrots dipped in leftover Sweet Cilantro Dressing

Dinner: Roasted Zucchini Pesto Lasagna Stacks (page 133) with Addictive Garlic-Roasted Broccoli (page 85)

BEGINNER
FIVE-DAY
SHOPPING LIST

FRESH PRODUCE

4 heads of romaine lettuce

1 head of butter lettuce

10 ounces fresh baby spinach

1 small head of cabbage or 2 (12-ounce) bags of shredded cabbage

1 large bunch fresh dill

1 large bunch fresh flat-leaf parsley

1 bunch fresh basil

1 bunch fresh cilantro

11 garlic cloves or 1 garlic bulb

2-inch knob of fresh ginger

1 jalapeño chile

2 large red onions

3 yellow onions

1 shallot

1 large bunch green onions

3 large cucumbers

4 carrots

8 red bell peppers

1 green bell pepper

1 pint cherry tomatoes

3 large tomatoes

1 large eggplant

3 pounds broccoli

2 zucchini

1 large parsnip

2 large sweet potatoes

1 (3-pound) spaghetti squash

3 Hass avocados

1 large navel orange

8 large lemons

10 to 15 olives, such as Castelvetrano

1 box Medjool dates (about 20 large dates)

1 lime

1 banana (plus more, optional, for snacks)

Assorted fresh fruit (optional, for snacks)

Assorted sliced veggies (optional, for snacks)

Mixed greens (optional, for side salads)

FROZEN ITEMS

1 (10-ounce) bag frozen mango chunks

1 (12-ounce) bag frozen artichoke hearts

ANIMAL PROTEIN

8 eggs

3 ounces goat cheddar (plus more, optional, for snacks)

8 ounces plain goat's milk yogurt

4 ounces goat feta cheese

4 ounces chèvre (soft goat cheese)

1 cup grated Pecorino Romano cheese

PANTRY STAPLES

2 cups raw walnuts

1 cup hulled pumpkin seeds

1 cup hulled sunflower seeds

1½ cups shredded unsweetened coconut

1 cup dried red lentils

3 cups quinoa

1 (28-ounce) box or jar tomato puree (strained tomatoes)

2 (15-ounce) cans black beans or dried black beans to cook

1 (15-ounce) can chickpeas or dried chickpeas to cook

Nondairy milk (optional, for serving with Nut-Free Gingerbread Granola)

4 to 6 sandwich rolls (or 4 to 6 sweet potatoes, for Sloppy Joe–Stuffed Sweet Potatoes)

6 to 8 burger buns (or large lettuce leaves, for Speedy Black Bean Burgers)

Gluten-free bread (optional)

SPEEDY MEAL PLAN

While I have developed all of the recipes in this book with ease and speed in mind, the following meal plan is designed to make a week's worth of healthy eating as fast as possible. I've included plenty of variety, but if you have leftovers one week, feel free to eat those to avoid spending extra time in the kitchen. Most of the recipes serve four people, aside from smoothies and skillets that serve only one or two, so be sure to adjust the meal plan and shopping list to fit your household's needs. With the exception of the Make It Ahead items, all of the breakfasts and lunches listed should come together in just about 10 minutes, and the dinners should take 30 minutes or less.

MAKE IT AHEAD OPTIONS

Butternut Stuffing · Cream of Buckwheat Porridge
Creamy Herb Dressing · Date Energy Bites · Freezer Oat Waffles
Mediterranean Quinoa Salad · Rainbow Lo Mein

MONDAY

Breakfast: Frosty Chocolate Shake (page 30)

Snack (optional): A ripe banana

Lunch: Mediterranean Quinoa Salad (page 66)

Snack (optional): Sliced cucumbers topped with sliced goat cheddar

Dinner: Pizza Stir-Fry (page 151) with side salad

TUESDAY

Breakfast: Orange-Mango Creamsicle Smoothie (page 34)

Snack (optional): A piece of fruit

Lunch: Creamy Kale Salad (page 65) and two Date Energy Bites (page 111)

Snack (optional): Sliced carrots or cucumbers

Dinner: Butternut Stuffing (page 144) with side salad

WEDNESDAY

Breakfast: Freezer Oat Waffles (page 49)

Snack (optional): A handful of raw nuts or seeds

Lunch: Chickpea & Avocado "Egg" Salad (page 61) on gluten-free bread

Snack (optional): Veggies dipped in Creamy Herb Dressing (page 56)

Dinner: Rainbow Lo Mein (page 147) with side salad

THURSDAY

Breakfast: Ginger Peach Detox Smoothie (page 33)

Snack (optional): A piece of fruit

Lunch: Leftover Mediterranean Quinoa Salad

Snack (optional): Sliced red bell peppers in Creamy Herb Dressing

Dinner: Mushroom & Black Bean Tacos with Avocado Crema (page 157)

FRIDAY

Breakfast: Cream of Buckwheat Porridge (page 39)

Snack (optional): A piece of fruit

Lunch: Shredded Brussels Sprout Salad (page 72)

Snack (optional): One Date Energy Bite

Dinner: One-Pot Quinoa Fried Rice (page 150) with side salad

SPEEDY SHOPPING LIST

FRESH PRODUCE

1 head of romaine lettuce

1 (3-pound) head of cabbage or preshredded cabbage

1½ pounds lacinato kale

2 cups fresh baby spinach

1 large bunch fresh dill

1 large bunch fresh flat-leaf parsley

1 large bunch fresh cilantro

1 small bunch fresh sage

1 small bunch fresh thyme

1 small bunch fresh chives

9 garlic cloves or 1 garlic bulb

3-inch knob of fresh ginger

4 red onions

3 yellow onions

1 large bunch green onions

6 celery stalks

5 red bell peppers

1 green bell pepper

1 small head of broccoli

1 pound brussels sprouts

2 zucchini

7 carrots

2 pounds whole or sliced cremini mushrooms

1 (2½-pound) butternut squash or 2 pounds precut cubes

1 large sweet potato

3 ripe Hass avocados

1 box Medjool dates (about 25 large dates)

7 large lemons

1 lime

1 large navel orange

1 banana (plus more, optional, for snacks)

10 to 15 olives, such as Castelvetrano

Assorted fresh fruit (optional, for snacks)

Assorted sliced veggies (optional, for snacks)

Mixed greens (optional, for side salads)

FROZEN ITEMS

1 (10-ounce) bag frozen mango chunks

1 (10-ounce) bag frozen peaches

1 (10-ounce) bag frozen strawberries

ANIMAL PROTEIN

4 ounces goat feta cheese

Raw goat cheddar (optional, for snacks)

¼ cup grated Pecorino Romano

PANTRY STAPLES

3 cups quinoa

1 cup raw buckwheat groats

1 (7-ounce) jar tomato paste (no salt added)

½ cup raisins

½ cup slivered almonds

2 cups walnuts

1 cup shredded unsweetened coconut

½ cup dried cranberries (optional)

½ cup chopped pecans (optional)

1 (15-ounce) can chickpeas or dried chickpeas to cook

1 (15-ounce) can black beans or dried black beans to cook

4 ounces brown rice spaghetti noodles

8 gluten-free tortillas (or butter lettuce leaves)

Nondairy milk (optional)

Gluten-free bread (optional)

BUDGET-FRIENDLY MEAL PLAN

The most expensive items in your shopping cart are usually animal products, including meat, dairy, and high-quality eggs, so this plan minimizes those expensive ingredients while still leaving you satisfied with plenty of plant-based protein. Each day of meals costs less than $6 per person, although keep in mind that costs may fluctuate depending on where you live. (All costs in this book were calculated using current grocery-store prices in the Midwest.) Most of these recipes will serve up to four people, so be sure to adjust your shopping list to fit your household's needs.

MAKE IT AHEAD OPTIONS

Creamy "Peanut" Dressing · Date Energy Bites · Freezer Oat Waffles
Knock-Off Italian Dressing · Mediterranean Quinoa Salad
Nut-Free Gingerbread Granola · Speedy Black Bean Burgers

MONDAY

Breakfast: Cream of Buckwheat Porridge (page 39) - $0.82

Snack (optional): A ripe banana - $0.19

Lunch: Chickpea & Avocado "Egg" Salad (page 61) - $1.58

Snack (optional): One Date Energy Bite (page 111) - $0.20

Dinner: Speedy Black Bean Burgers (page 130) - $0.71 - with a side salad - $0.83

Total: $4.33 per person

TUESDAY

Breakfast: Freezer Oat Waffles (page 49) - $1.30

Snack (optional): An apple - $0.50

Lunch: Creamy Kale Salad (page 65) - $1.30

Snack (optional): Sliced veggies - $0.30

Dinner: Sloppy Joe–Stuffed Sweet Potatoes (page 118) - $1.39 - with side salad - $0.83

Total: $5.62 per person

WEDNESDAY

Breakfast: Frozen Chai Latte (page 37) - $1.21

Snack (optional): A ripe banana - $0.19

Lunch: Crunchy Thai Salad with Creamy "Peanut" Dressing (page 70) - $1.63

Snack (optional): One Date Energy Bite - $0.20

Dinner: Mexican Quinoa Stew (page 83) - $1.46 - with side salad - $0.83

Total: $5.52 per person

THURSDAY

Breakfast: Skillet Breakfast Hash (page 50) - $0.89

Snack (optional): A handful of raw almonds - $0.50

Lunch: Southwest Lettuce Wraps with Sweet Cilantro Dressing (page 104) - $1.71

Snack (optional): Sliced veggies with leftover Creamy "Peanut" Dressing - $0.30

Dinner: Butternut Mac 'n' Cheese (page 122) - $1.23 - with side salad - $0.83

Total: $5.46 per person

FRIDAY

Breakfast: Nut-Free Gingerbread Granola (page 38) - $0.99 - with rice milk - $0.11

Snack (optional): A ripe banana - $0.19

Lunch: Mediterranean Quinoa Salad (page 66) - $1.86

Snack (optional): One Date Energy Bite - $0.20

Dinner: Vegan Shepherd's Pie (page 134) - $1.46 - with side salad - $0.83

Total: $5.64 per person

BUDGET-FRIENDLY SHOPPING LIST

NOTE: Stocking your pantry with dry bulk items such as almond butter, chia seeds, and raw cacao powder can be pricey at first, but keep in mind that these items should last for several months, so subsequent visits to the store will be much cheaper.

FRESH PRODUCE

2 heads of romaine lettuce

1 head of butter lettuce

2 cups fresh baby spinach (optional)

1 head of cabbage or 2 (12-ounce) bags of shredded cabbage

1 pound lacinato kale

1 large bunch fresh cilantro

2 large bunches fresh flat-leaf parsley

1 large bunch fresh dill

1 small bunch fresh chives

1 small bunch fresh rosemary

1 small bunch fresh thyme

14 garlic cloves or 1 garlic bulb

2-inch knob of fresh ginger

1 large bunch green onions

3 jalapeño chiles

3 red onions

4 yellow onions

2 green bell peppers

5 red bell peppers

2 cucumbers

4 celery stalks

12 carrots

2 cups fresh shelled English peas (or frozen)

8 ounces whole or sliced cremini mushrooms

2½ pounds sweet potatoes

1 (1½-pound) butternut squash or 1 pound frozen cubes

3 Hass avocados

1 large lime

6 large lemons

1 box Medjool dates (about 21 large dates)

10 to 15 olives, such as Castelvetrano

Assorted fresh fruit (optional, for snacks)

Assorted sliced veggies (optional, for snacks)

Mixed greens (optional, for side salads)

ANIMAL PROTEIN

4 eggs

2 ounces raw goat cheddar

¼ cup grated Pecorino Romano cheese

PANTRY STAPLES

2 cups walnuts

1 cup hulled pumpkin seeds

1 cup hulled sunflower seeds

1½ cups shredded unsweetened coconut

½ cup raisins

½ cup slivered almonds

2½ cups quinoa

1 cup raw buckwheat groats

1¾ cups dried red lentils

1 (15-ounce) can chickpeas or dried chickpeas to cook

3 (15-ounce) cans black beans or dried black beans to cook

1 (28-ounce) box or jar chopped tomatoes

1 (28-ounce) box or jar tomato puree (strained tomatoes)

6 to 8 high-quality burger buns (or large butter lettuce leaves for Speedy Black Bean Burgers)

4 to 6 sandwich buns (or sweet potatoes, for Sloppy Joe-Stuffed Sweet Potatoes)

1 pound gluten-free macaroni or shell pasta

Raw almonds (optional, for snacks)

Nondairy milk (optional, for Nut-Free Gingerbread Granola)

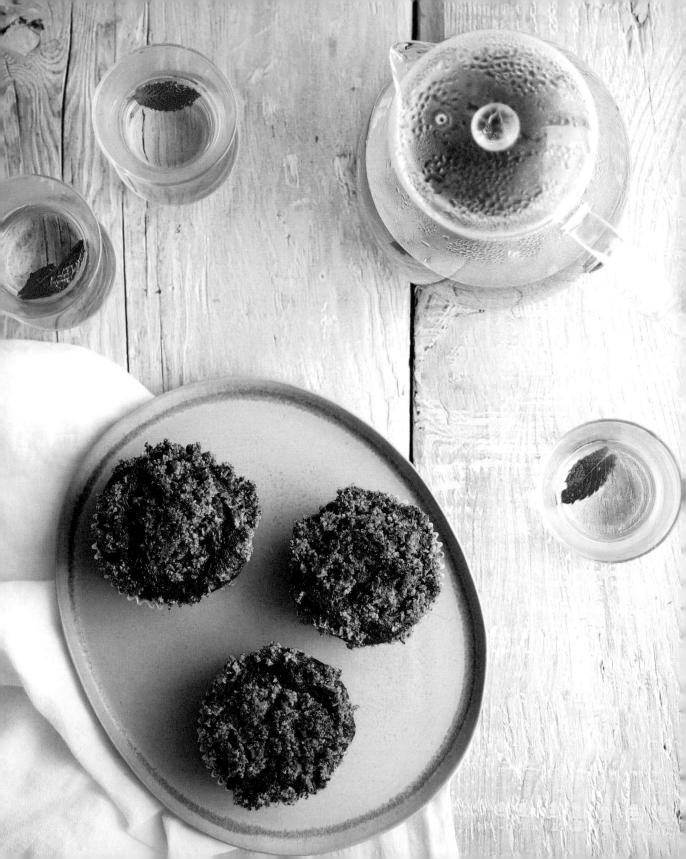

2 SPEEDY SHAKES & MORNING FAVORITES

frosty chocolate shake

SERVES 1 | $3.39 PER SERVING

NUT/SEED/DRIED FRUIT

DF EF GF NS V

1 cup water

2 tablespoons chia seeds

1½ tablespoons raw cacao powder

1 tablespoon raw cashew butter

1 teaspoon vanilla extract

Large handful of fresh baby spinach

4 or 5 soft Medjool dates, pitted (see Note)

1½ to 2 cups ice cubes

This creamy chocolate shake is one of my go-to breakfasts, and is also one of the most-requested desserts in my home. Rather than relying on a frozen banana, which is often used in frosty smoothie recipes, this shake is naturally sweetened with juicy dates to avoid impacting the chocolatey flavor. Dates are one of my favorite low-glycemic sweeteners because they contain essential minerals such as calcium, iron, and magnesium, while providing a neutral sweet flavor and plenty of fiber. If you don't have a high-speed blender, soak the dates and chia seeds in the water for 20 minutes before blending, or even overnight in the fridge, to help them break down more smoothly.

1 Combine the water, chia seeds, cacao powder, cashew butter, vanilla, spinach, and 4 of the dates in a high-speed blender and blend until completely smooth. Taste the mixture and adjust any ingredients, adding the remaining date if more sweetness is desired. (Keep in mind that adding the ice in the next step will dilute the flavor a bit.)

2 Add in 1½ cups of the ice cubes and blend until an ice cream–like consistency is achieved, adding more ice if needed. Serve immediately.

MAKE IT NUT-FREE: You can replace the cashew butter with Sunflower Butter (page 187) or raw tahini for a nut-free shake.

NOTE: If another type of date, like Deglet, is easier to find, keep in mind that many dates are smaller than Medjool, and you'll need to double the amount to make this shake sweet enough. Dates are a low-glycemic fruit and are considered a healthy addition to a type 2 diabetes diet,[1] and as an added bonus, studies have shown that eating six dates a day may help pregnant women have easier deliveries, too.[2] (I can attest to that fact myself!)

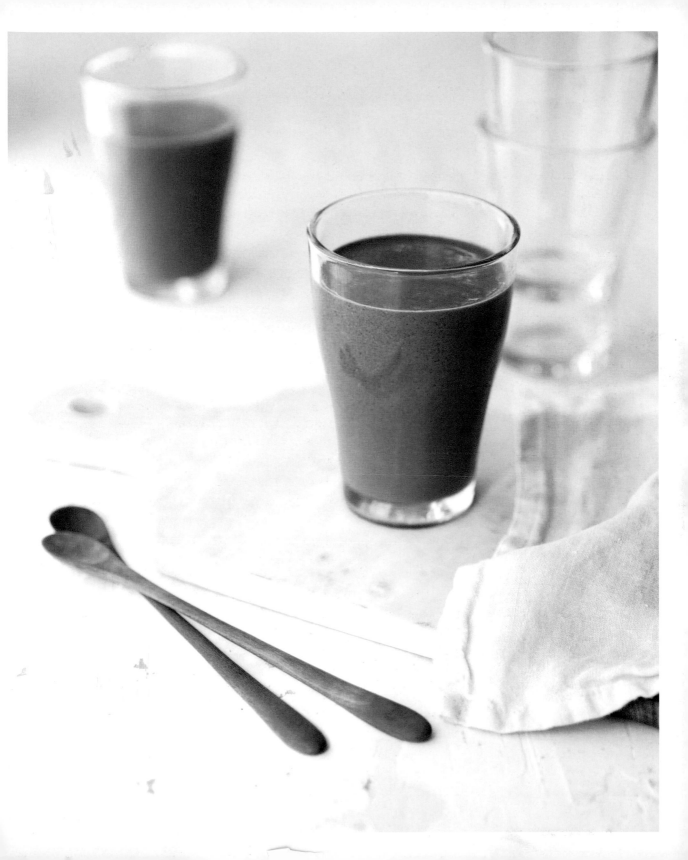

sweet tart smoothie

SERVES 1 | $4.19 PER SERVING

FRESH FRUIT

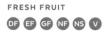

1 cup coconut water
(see Note)

1 cup frozen raspberries

1 cup frozen mango
chunks

1 cup fresh pineapple
chunks

2 soft Medjool dates,
pitted

This smoothie is inspired by the popular childhood candies that have a refreshingly sweet and tart flavor. Using coconut water as the base, this shake packs a healthy dose of electrolytes to energize your morning, along with 25 percent of the needed daily value for vitamin A from the added mango. This powerful vitamin not only helps with night vision but also helps your skin repel bacteria and viruses more effectively, making this shake a delicious way to boost your immune system.

1   Combine all of the ingredients in a high-speed blender and blend until smooth. Taste and adjust any of the flavors. Serve immediately.

NOTE: For best flavor, use fresh coconut water from a young Thai coconut or a bottled coconut water that is labeled as "raw." I've listed my favorite brands in Resources on page 192.

ginger peach detox smoothie

SERVES 1 | $2.70 PER SERVING

30-MINUTE RECIPE

Ginger and peach make a natural pair, and when you add in a handful of strawberries and cilantro, you have a powerful antioxidant-rich and detoxifying drink, too. Cilantro is helpful in pulling heavy metals out of the body, but start with a very small amount, since it can cause a "detox headache" if you do too much too soon. A little bit goes a long way with fresh ginger, too. If you're not a big ginger fan, I recommend starting with no more than the size of the very tip of your pinkie finger so that it doesn't overwhelm the other flavors in your shake.

FRESH FRUIT
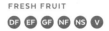

1 cup water

1½ cups frozen peaches

5 frozen strawberries

1 tablespoon freshly squeezed lemon juice

¼ ripe Hass avocado

2 or 3 soft Medjool dates, pitted

½ to 1 teaspoon minced fresh ginger

2 to 3 tablespoons chopped fresh cilantro

1   Combine all of the ingredients in a blender, starting with just 2 of the dates, ½ teaspoon of the ginger, and 2 tablespoons of the cilantro and blend until smooth. Taste and add the remaining date and more ginger or cilantro, if desired. Serve immediately.

Don't Fear Fruit

The idea that "sugar is sugar" in the body is a common misconception among the health community, but research has shown that the sugar in fruit does not impact the body the same way industrial fructose does. In fact, fruit may actually blunt insulin spikes! In one study, fruit was blended into an already sugary beverage. Even though the added fruit increased the overall sugar content of the drink, participants drinking it were found to have a lower insulin spike when compared to those drinking the sugary beverage on its own.[3] Another small study showed that even when subjects consumed a whopping twenty servings of fruit each day, there was no adverse effects on their body weight, blood pressure, insulin, or lipid levels, despite the high fructose intake.[4] Research published in 2013 concluded that fruit should not even be restricted in patients with type 2 diabetes.[5] If weight loss is your goal, a moderate-fructose diet has been shown to be more effective than a low-fructose diet, too.[6] While there are always exceptions to the rule, I hope that the general population will not fear fruit and risk missing out on its valuable nutrition.

orange-mango creamsicle smoothie

SERVES 1 | $2.19 PER SERVING

FRESH FRUIT

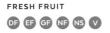

½ cup water

½ large orange, peeled with any seeds removed

½ frozen banana

1 heaping cup frozen mango chunks

¼ ripe Hass avocado

Large handful of fresh baby spinach

This smoothie is always a crowd-pleaser and tastes like refreshing tropical ice cream. My son actually calls it "green ice cream" and will enjoy it for breakfast, as an afternoon snack, or as a dessert. The antioxidants found in oranges and mangoes are thought to lower cholesterol and may help with blood sugar regulation,[7] so it's a creamy treat that you can feel good about indulging in regularly.

1   Combine all of the ingredients in a high-speed blender and blend until smooth and creamy, adding more water if needed to facilitate blending. Serve immediately.

NOTE: When you freeze your bananas, make sure they have lots of brown spots on their skin; this will ensure that they are sweet and ripe. Peel the banana before freezing it, or the skin will never come off. If you don't have a powerful blender, try slicing the banana into ½-inch coins and freezing for easier blending.

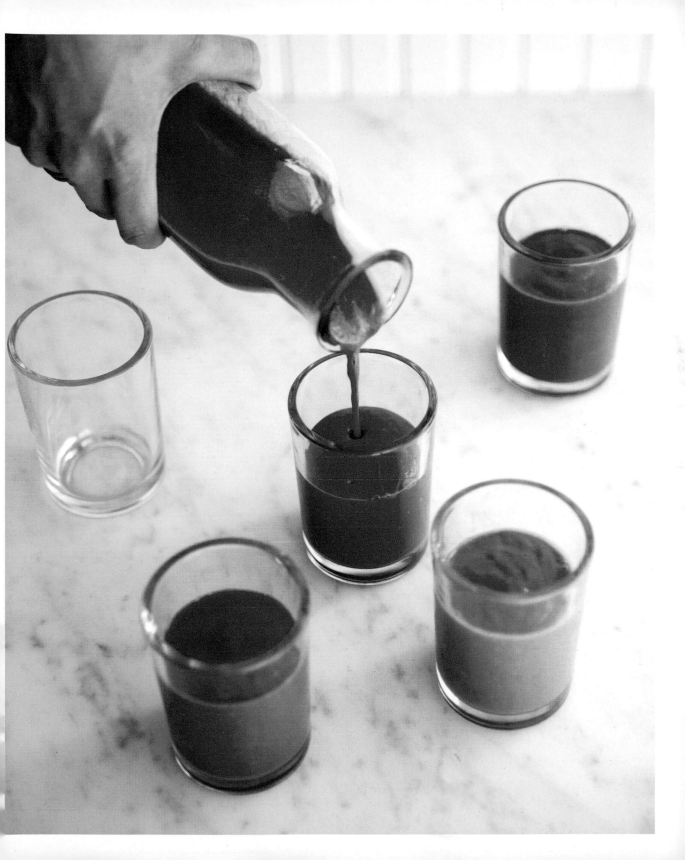

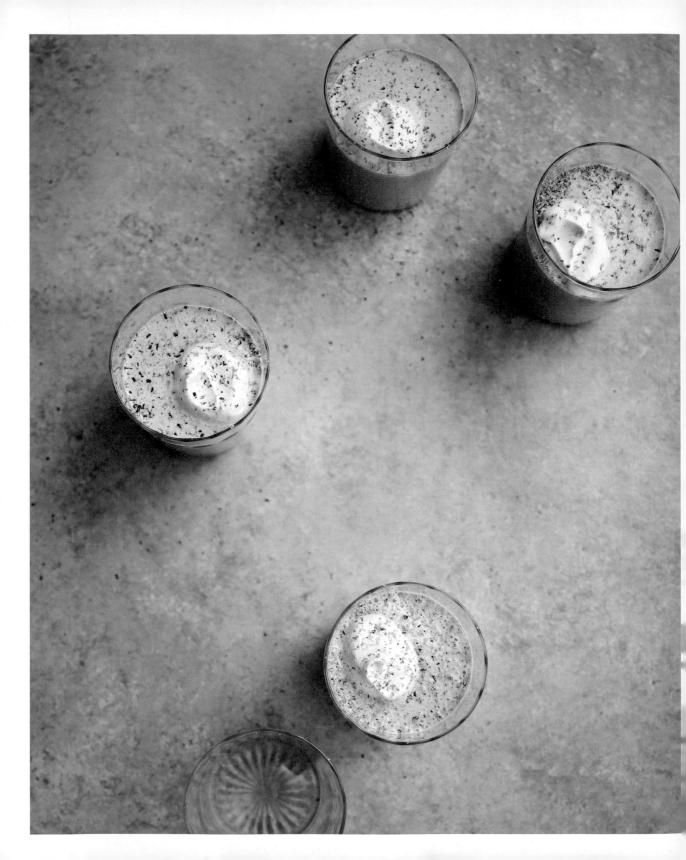

frozen chai latte

SERVES 1 | $1.21 PER SERVING

This smoothie is another family favorite. The flavor reminds me of a frozen chai latte, but this recipe is better than any coffeehouse version because it's caffeine-free and loaded with heart-healthy superseeds. Tahini is bursting with calcium, hemp hearts are loaded with complete protein, and flax seeds are brimming with omega-3 fatty acids for a shake that will keep you satisfied all morning long. Top with a dollop of Coconut Cream (page 184) if you like.

1   Combine the water, flax seeds, hemp hearts, tahini, cinnamon, ginger, nutmeg, and 4 of the dates in a high-speed blender and blend until smooth. (At this point the texture will be thick and pudding-like, but it's a good time to taste for sweetness and add the remaining date, if necessary.)

2   Add in the ice and blend until thick and creamy. Taste and adjust any flavors as needed. Serve immediately.

NOTE: If you don't have a high-speed blender, be sure to combine the smoothie ingredients (except for the ice) at least 15 minutes ahead of time, or even overnight, to help the dates and seeds soften and break down more easily.

NUT/SEED/DRIED FRUIT

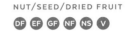

1 cup water

1 tablespoon ground flax seeds

1 tablespoon hemp hearts

1 tablespoon raw tahini

¼ teaspoon ground cinnamon

¼ teaspoon ground ginger

Pinch of nutmeg

4 or 5 soft Medjool dates, pitted

1 (16-ounce) glass ice cubes

nut-free gingerbread granola

SERVES 4 | $0.99 PER SERVING

NUT/SEED/DRIED FRUIT

(DF) (EF) (GF) (NF) (NS) (V)

1 cup hulled pumpkin seeds

½ cup hulled sunflower seeds

½ cup shredded unsweetened coconut

1 teaspoon ground cinnamon

½ teaspoon ground ginger

⅛ teaspoon fine sea salt

¼ cup maple syrup

2 teaspoons blackstrap molasses

The cereal aisle is filled with colorful boxes of iron-fortified cereals that are often loaded with sugar and empty carbs, so this granola is my healthier alternative. It's naturally sweetened with mineral-rich maple syrup and has blackstrap molasses added for a boost of iron. I always associate molasses with gingerbread cookies, so the flavor of this grain-free cereal reminds me of a cross between gingerbread cookies and a chai latte. Enjoy it with your favorite nondairy milk or yogurt for a satiating breakfast or snack.

1   Preheat the oven to 250°F and line a large baking sheet with parchment paper. Place the pumpkin seeds in a food processor fitted with an "S" blade and briefly pulse, just enough to break the seeds down into smaller pieces but leaving a few chunks for texture in the granola.

2   Transfer the pulsed seeds to a large mixing bowl and add in the rest of the ingredients. Stir well until all of the seeds are evenly coated with the syrup and spices.

3   Spread the mixture onto the prepared baking sheet and use a spatula to spread it into a thin, even layer. The thinner it is, the crispier it will get.

4   Bake until the granola no longer feels wet to the touch, about 40 minutes. Allow to cool completely; the granola will become crispy as it cools.

5   Break the granola into small chunks and store in an airtight container at room temperature for up to 4 days or in the refrigerator for up to 2 weeks.

cream of buckwheat porridge

SERVES 4 | $0.82 PER SERVING

If you grew up eating Cream of Wheat as I did, this porridge is a satisfying gluten-free alternative to that childhood favorite. Despite its name, buckwheat isn't at all related to wheat and is actually a gluten-free seed that is a great source of easily digestible protein. While buckwheat flour can be bitter, the raw groats have a mild, nutty flavor and cook significantly faster when ground ahead of time, making this breakfast a real time-saver on busy mornings.

STARCH

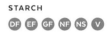

1   Grind the groats in a coffee grinder or high-speed blender until a fine meal is created, about 10 seconds. It's okay if there are still a few chunks. (You may need to do this ½ cup at a time if using a small coffee grinder.)

2   Using a large whisk, combine the ground groats, water, and cinnamon in a small saucepan. (It's important to use cold water to start with, as hot water will cause the groats to clump.)

3   Place the saucepan on the stove over medium-high heat and bring the cereal to a boil. Use the whisk to stir as the cereal boils, then lower the heat to a simmer and let the cereal cook until thickened and tender, about 10 minutes. Stir occasionally to make sure the bottom isn't burning.

4   Season with the salt and maple syrup, then serve warm with a splash of nondairy milk.

MAKE IT AHEAD: This cooked cereal will keep well in an airtight container in the refrigerator for up to 1 week, so feel free to make a large batch ahead of time and store it in individual serving containers. It's even tasty cold.

1 cup raw buckwheat groats

4 cups cold water

2 teaspoons ground cinnamon

Pinch of fine sea salt

¼ cup maple syrup

Nondairy milk, for serving (optional)

morning glory snack muffins

MAKES 12 MUFFINS | $0.47 PER MUFFIN

SPECIAL TREAT

(DF) (GF) (NF) (NS)

2 large ripe bananas

¾ cup coconut flour

6 eggs, at room temperature

½ cup coconut sugar

¼ cup coconut oil, melted

1 teaspoon vanilla extract

1 teaspoon ground cinnamon

1 teaspoon baking soda

½ teaspoon fine sea salt

1½ cups tightly packed shredded carrots

½ cup raisins

These muffins are a great way to sneak more veggies into a picky eater's diet, without tasting "healthy" at all. I decreased some of the sugar found in traditional muffins by using naturally sweet bananas and carrots, while a sprinkling of raisins and cinnamon makes these muffins taste like a bakery treat. Loaded with protein and fiber, they make an easy, filling breakfast or portable snack.

1   Preheat the oven to 350°F and line a standard muffin tin with 12 baking cups (see Note).

2   In a large mixing bowl, mash the bananas, then add the coconut flour, eggs, coconut sugar, coconut oil, vanilla, cinnamon, baking soda, and salt. Stir well to combine. (If your eggs are cold, don't be surprised if this mixture is very thick, since the coconut oil will firm up when mixed with cold ingredients. That shouldn't affect the final texture; it just makes the mixing process slightly more difficult.)

3   Once a uniform batter is created, fold in the carrots and raisins and then divide the batter among the prepared muffin cups.

4   Bake for 25 to 30 minutes, until the edges are golden and the centers are firm to the touch. Allow the muffins to cool completely before serving. Store leftover muffins in an airtight container in the refrigerator for up to 1 week, or in the freezer for up to 3 months. When you're ready to serve, thaw at room temperature, which can take up to 4 hours, or in the refrigerator overnight.

NOTE: I prefer to use silicone baking cups when baking with eggs or coconut flour because the silicone seems to offer the absolute best stick prevention. Most parchment baking cups are lined with silicone anyway, but I find that the silicone cups work even better in comparison.

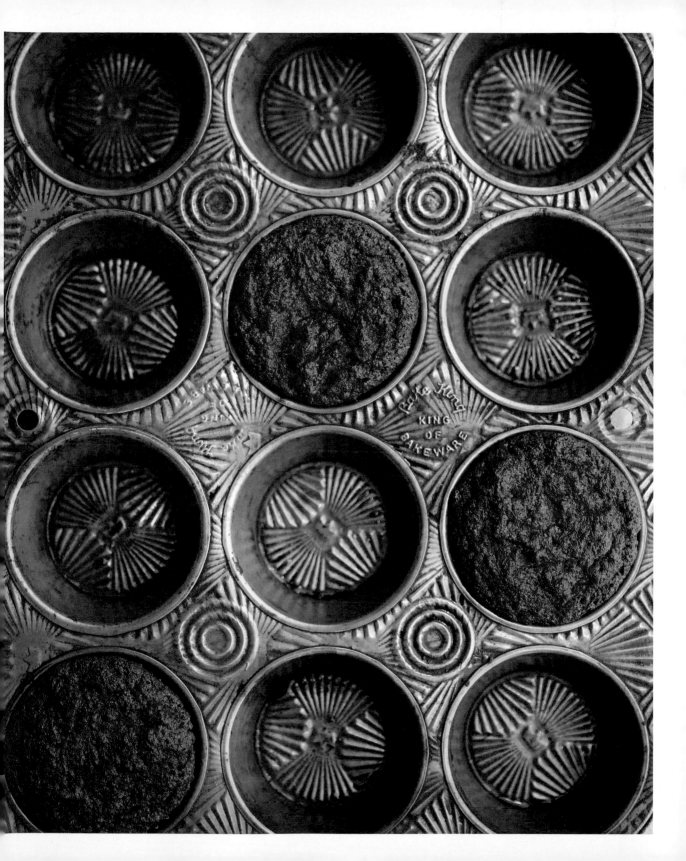

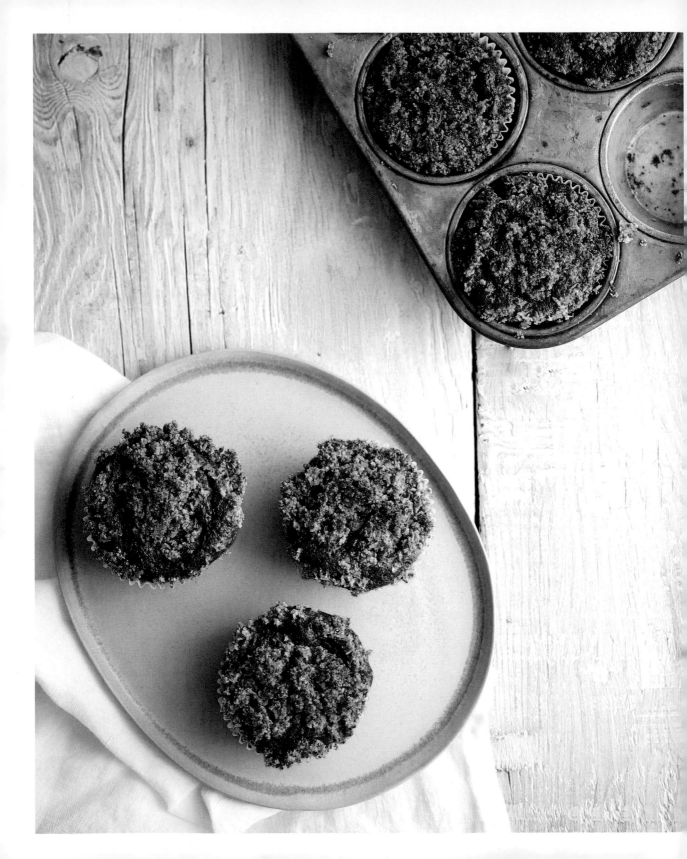

cashew butter spice muffins

MAKES 12 MUFFINS | $0.66 PER MUFFIN

These gluten-free muffins are so unbelievably light and fluffy that no one will believe they are made without the use of flour or refined sugar. Don't be deceived by their light texture, though—these nutrient-dense muffins are still very filling, thanks to the healthful fat found in cashews and protein-rich eggs. Topped with a buttery crumble, they are hard to resist.

SPECIAL TREAT

1   Preheat the oven to 350°F and line a standard muffin tin with 12 baking cups.

2   To prepare the batter: In a large mixing bowl, combine the cashew butter, coconut sugar, applesauce, eggs, baking soda, salt, cinnamon, ginger, and nutmeg and stir well to create a smooth, runny batter. Divide the batter among the prepared baking cups.

3   To prepare the crumble: In a small food processor, combine the cashews, shredded coconut, coconut sugar, and salt and process until coarsely ground. Add the coconut oil and process again until the mixture starts to stick together.

4   Sprinkle the crumble over the top of the batter in each baking cup and press lightly on the top to make sure the crumble will stick to the baked muffin.

5   Bake the muffins for about 20 minutes, until the tops are firm and lightly golden. Allow to cool completely before serving. Store leftover muffins in an airtight container in the refrigerator for up to 1 week, or in the freezer for up to 3 months. When you're ready to serve, thaw at room temperature, which can take up to 4 hours, or in the refrigerator overnight.

NOTE: While many nuts and seeds are susceptible to acrylamide formation when exposed to high temperatures (see page 103), cashews seem to be an exception to the rule, with no acrylamide detected when they are roasted.[8] That is the reason these muffins and the Deep-Dish Chocolate Chip Cookie on page 163 are not baked at a lower temperature the way the rest of my nut-based recipes are. There's no need to wait any longer than you have to for these delicious baked goods to be ready.

BATTER

1 cup creamy cashew butter

½ cup coconut sugar

½ cup unsweetened applesauce

2 eggs, beaten

½ teaspoon baking soda

¼ teaspoon fine sea salt

2 teaspoons ground cinnamon

½ teaspoon ground ginger

¼ teaspoon ground nutmeg

CRUMBLE

½ cup raw cashews

¼ cup shredded unsweetened coconut

2 tablespoons coconut sugar

Pinch of fine sea salt

2 tablespoons coconut oil, melted

broccoli cheddar egg muffins

MAKES 12 MUFFINS | $0.50 PER MUFFIN

ANIMAL PROTEIN

1 tablespoon butter
or coconut oil

3 cups chopped
broccoli, chopped
as finely as possible

½ yellow onion,
chopped

4 eggs, beaten

½ cup water

¾ teaspoon fine
sea salt

3 ounces goat cheddar,
shredded

Quichelike—without a crust—these egg-based muffins are an easy protein-packed option to grab on the go. I like to chop the broccoli finely so that it's evenly distributed in each bite; this helps make the texture more appealing to picky eaters, too. Broccoli and cheddar have always been a classic match, so these muffins are a great way to squeeze in a serving of veggies at the very start of your day. They even work great for lunch or dinner.

1   Preheat the oven to 350°F and line a standard muffin tin with 12 baking cups (see Note, page 40).

2   In a 10-inch skillet, melt the butter over medium heat. Add the broccoli and onion and sauté until tender, 6 to 8 minutes.

3   In a large mixing bowl, beat together the eggs, water, and salt and stir in the cheese. Add the veggies to the mix and stir well. Divide the batter among the prepared baking cups.

4   Bake until the eggs are set, about 30 minutes. Serve warm. Store leftover muffins in an airtight container in the refrigerator for up to 1 week.

mushroom & leek egg bake

SERVES 4 TO 6 | $1.31 TO $1.97 PER SERVING

Although this dish is technically a frittata, the number of veggies stuffed into it gives it more of a quichelike texture. In fact, the spaghetti squash strands go almost unnoticed—my own mother thought it was just cheese! This baked egg dish is a great way to sneak more vegetables into your morning with plenty of protein to keep you satisfied, although you could enjoy it with a leafy green salad at any time of the day. It comes together rather quickly if you cook the spaghetti squash ahead of time (see page 14).

1   Preheat the oven to 350°F and generously grease a 10-inch pie pan.

2   Melt the butter in a large skillet or Dutch oven and sauté the leeks until wilted and tender, about 8 minutes. Add the mushrooms and ¼ teaspoon of the salt and cook until the mushrooms shrink in size and release their moisture, about 8 minutes more. Add the cooked squash and stir well to combine. (If your spaghetti squash is cold from being in the refrigerator, be sure to sauté again until it is heated through.)

3   In a large mixing bowl, whisk together the eggs, Pecorino Romano, and remaining ½ teaspoon salt. Add the cooked veggies, then pour the mixture into the prepared pie pan. Sprinkle the shredded cheddar over the top.

4   Bake for about 35 minutes, until the center is set and the top is lightly golden. (The center may rise with baking, but it will later deflate when you remove it from the oven.) Allow to cool for 10 minutes before slicing and serving. Store leftovers in an airtight container in the refrigerator for up to 4 days.

NOTE: Be sure to cut the leeks down the middle and rinse well before slicing, since leeks usually contain lots of dirt in their crevices. You don't want any dirt or residue in your final dish.

ANIMAL PROTEIN

1 teaspoon butter or coconut oil

2 leeks, white and light green parts, thinly sliced (see Note)

8 ounces mushrooms, coarsely chopped

¾ teaspoon fine sea salt

½ spaghetti squash, cooked

4 eggs, beaten

½ cup grated Pecorino Romano or Parmesan cheese

1 ounce goat cheddar, shredded

vegan pumpkin bread

MAKES 1 STANDARD LOAF | $0.62 PER SLICE

STARCH

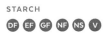

1½ cups gluten-free oat flour (see page 189)

1 cup pumpkin puree

1 cup coconut sugar

1 tablespoon ground cinnamon

¼ teaspoon ground ginger

¼ teaspoon ground cloves

¼ cup coconut oil, melted

1 teaspoon vanilla extract

1 teaspoon baking soda

¼ teaspoon fine sea salt

1 tablespoon raw apple cider vinegar

The vegan Buckwheat Pumpkin Bread on my website is wildly popular, but since the taste of buckwheat can be off-putting to many people, I wanted to come up with a more crowd-pleasing alternative. This quick bread recipe uses oat flour, without any additional gums or starches, to make it as easy as possible to whip up. Beware of making substitutions with this vegan and gluten-free recipe, since any change might affect the outcome. While it doesn't bake up as tall as a normal wheat-based loaf, it's super-moist and addictive.

1   Preheat the oven to 350°F and line a standard loaf pan with parchment paper.

2   In a large mixing bowl, combine the flour, pumpkin puree, coconut sugar, cinnamon, ginger, cloves, coconut oil, vanilla, baking soda, and salt and stir well to combine. Add the vinegar, and stir quickly to make sure it's fully incorporated.

3   Transfer the batter to the prepared loaf pan and use a spatula to spread it evenly into the bottom of the pan and smooth the top.

4   Bake until the center of the loaf is beginning to crack and feels firm to the touch, about 45 minutes. Allow to cool completely before removing from the pan and cutting. Store in an airtight container in the refrigerator for up to 1 week, or in the freezer for up to 3 months. When you're ready to serve, thaw at room temperature, which can take up to 4 hours, or in the refrigerator overnight.

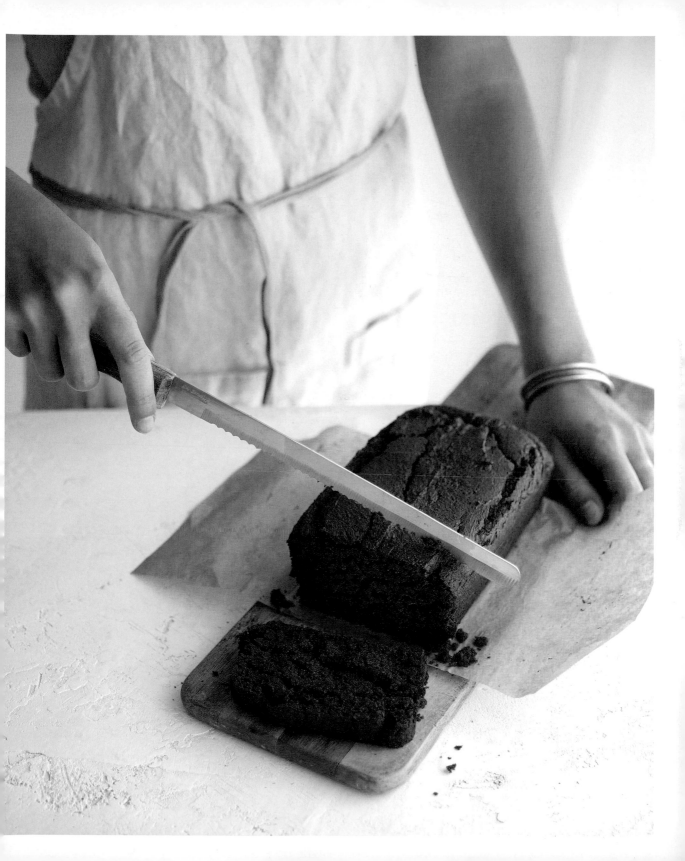

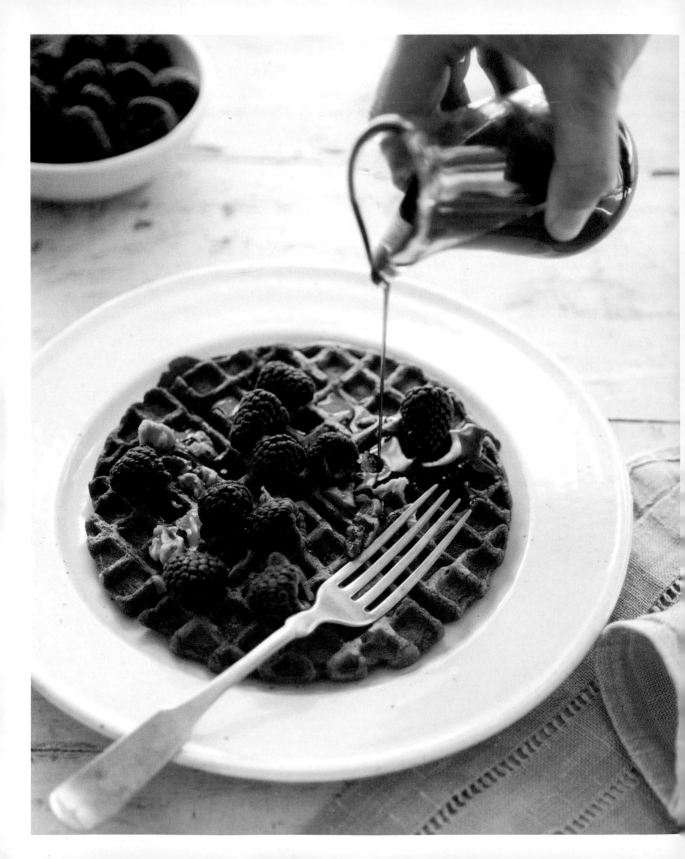

freezer oat waffles

MAKES 4 OR 5 CLASSIC WAFFLES OR 2 BELGIAN WAFFLES | $1.30 PER WAFFLE

These waffles are the perfect make-ahead breakfast because they reheat easily in a toaster, just like the popular freezer waffles I grew up with. I love sneaking an extra serving of vitamin-rich sweet potato into these crispy waffles, so feel free to double or triple this recipe to keep your freezer well stocked. Do not be tempted to try this recipe for pancakes. It simply doesn't work well without a waffle iron, and the result is a very flat pancake with a dense, gooey center.

STARCH

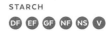

1. Generously grease your waffle iron with coconut oil, then preheat it according to the manufacturer's instructions.

2. In a large bowl, combine the flour, water, sweet potato, cinnamon, maple syrup, ¼ cup coconut oil, salt, baking soda, and vinegar and use a whisk to stir well. (Using a whisk will help you avoid any clumps.) Allow the batter to sit while the waffle iron preheats—the batter will thicken the longer it rests.

3. Pour about ¾ cup of the batter into the preheated waffle maker. (This amount should fill a classic-size waffle maker. If you have a Belgian-style waffle maker, more batter will be necessary since those waffles are much bigger, but keep in mind that they won't fit into a standard toaster for reheating later.)

4. Cook the waffles according to the manufacturer's instructions. (It's not unusual for these waffles to take several minutes longer to cook than traditional waffle batter, and you may see steam release from the waffle maker, which is also normal.) Continue to cook until the outside is crisp and dry to the touch, and the waffle is easily released from the waffle iron. The resulting waffle should be crisp on the outside and tender on the inside. Serve immediately. To freeze, store cooled waffles in an airtight container with a piece of parchment paper between each waffle to prevent sticking for up to 3 months. The frozen waffles can be cooked directly from the freezer in a toaster for a quick meal or snack.

¼ cup coconut oil, melted, plus more for greasing the waffle iron

2 cups gluten-free oat flour (see page 189)

1¾ cups water

1 cup mashed sweet potato

2 teaspoons ground cinnamon

¼ cup maple syrup

½ teaspoon fine sea salt

1 teaspoon baking soda

1 tablespoon raw apple cider vinegar

skillet breakfast hash

SERVES 2 | $0.89 PER SERVING

GF NF NS SF

1 tablespoon butter
or coconut oil

½ red onion, diced

½ green bell pepper,
diced

½ small head of green
cabbage, shredded

¼ teaspoon fine
sea salt

Freshly ground black
pepper

4 eggs

2 ounces raw goat
cheddar, shredded
(optional)

Freshly chopped chives,
for garnish

I developed this recipe for my dad, because one of his favorite breakfasts is "smothered and covered" hash browns (if you've ever been to Waffle House, you know what I'm talking about), served with eggs on top. Shredded cabbage makes the perfect substitute for hash browns, because it becomes tender like potatoes but is much lower in carbs while still being loaded with essential vitamins and minerals for a more nutrient-dense meal. Be sure to use the largest skillet you have when making this dish because the shredded cabbage is bulky at first but will soon shrink as it cooks. This is a one-pan meal if you bake the eggs in an oven, but you're welcome to cook the eggs in a separate skillet if you prefer.

1   Preheat the oven to 400°F. In a large, deep skillet over medium heat, melt the butter and sauté the onion and bell pepper until they start to soften, about 5 minutes. Add the cabbage, salt, and a few grinds of black pepper and cook until everything is tender, about 10 minutes more.

2   Crack the eggs into the skillet directly on top of the cooked vegetables, sprinkle with the cheese, and bake until the whites are cooked, 5 to 10 minutes. If you prefer runny yolks, check on the eggs starting at 5 minutes to avoid overcooking; for firmer yolks, cook for the entire 10 minutes. Serve warm, garnished with a sprinkling of fresh chives.

Why Is Goat's Milk Better?
Goat's milk is often thought of as a hypoallergenic alternative to cow's milk, as its protein structure is significantly different, containing less of the allergenic alpha S1 casein protein. Goat's milk has been studied as a substitute for cow's milk for children, and over a five-month period, those receiving goat's milk excelled in weight gain, height, and nutrition, when compared to children on cow's milk. In studies of children with allergies to cow's milk, treatment with goat's milk produced positive results in 93 percent of subjects, which also suggests that goat's milk is easier to digest and less allergenic.[9] Since goat's and sheep's milks are structurally similar, feel free to enjoy them both as an alternative to cow dairy.

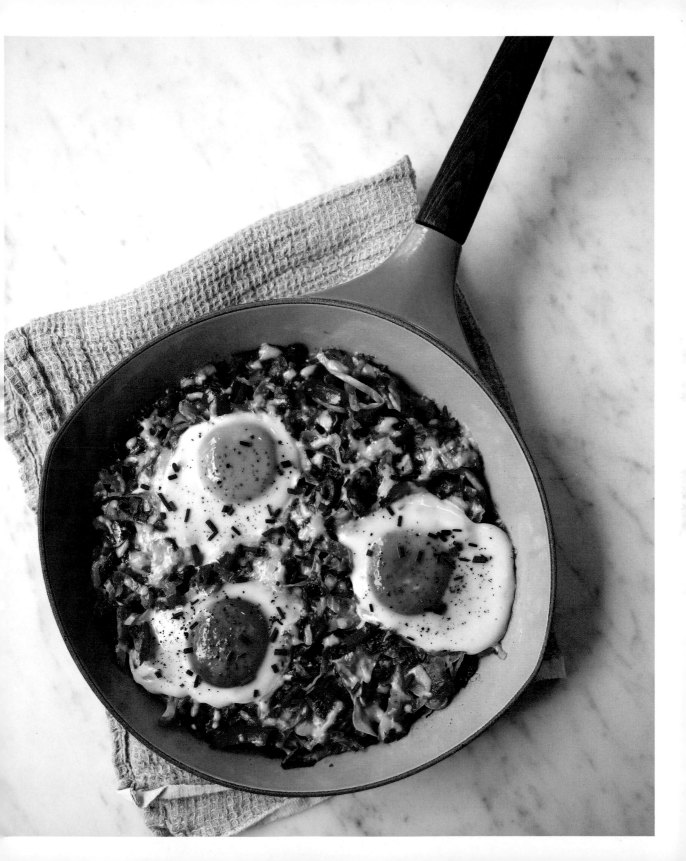

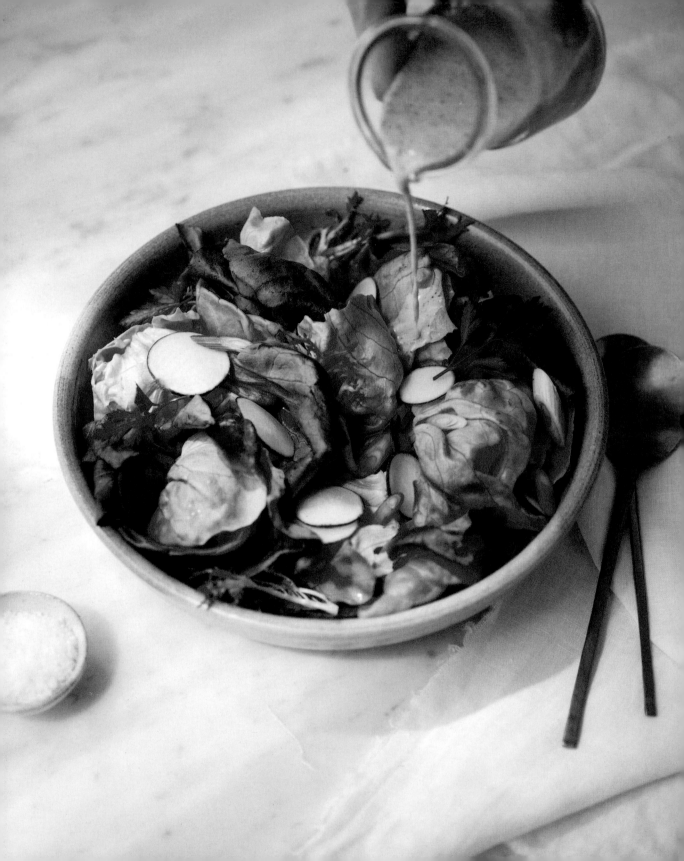

3 SALADS & DRESSINGS

knock-off italian dressing

MAKES ABOUT 1½ CUPS | $0.23 PER SERVING

ANIMAL PROTEIN

(EF) (GF) (NF) (NS)

⅔ cup extra-virgin olive oil

¼ cup raw apple cider vinegar

¼ cup water

2 cloves garlic

¾ teaspoon fine sea salt

¼ teaspoon freshly ground black pepper

1 teaspoon dried basil

½ teaspoon raw honey

¼ cup grated Pecorino Romano cheese

This salad dressing is reminiscent of one served at a popular Italian restaurant chain that serves unlimited salad and bread sticks. One thing that sets that particular salad dressing apart is the addition of grated cheese—it makes the dressing extra-creamy and salty, which is perfectly balanced over a pile of hydrating vegetables. I've kept the use of cheese to a minimum in this dressing, but the result will still leave you wanting a salad refill.

1   In a blender, combine all of the ingredients and blend until emulsified. You can serve immediately, but the flavor gets even better the longer it chills in the refrigerator. Store leftovers in an airtight container in the refrigerator for up to 5 days.

balsamic thyme vinaigrette

MAKES ABOUT 1 CUP | $0.34 PER SERVING

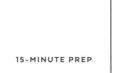

Balsamic vinegar is a flavorful addition to any favorite salad, and studies have shown that the acetic acid it contains may help improve blood glucose levels and lower blood pressure.[1] To help reduce the oil content, this dressing is blended with shallot and honey to help thicken it, and the addition of fresh thyme and rosemary will take the taste of your salad to the next level. I hope you enjoy the flavor over any number of salad combinations.

NEUTRAL

¼ cup balsamic vinegar

1½ tablespoons raw honey

1 clove garlic

1 teaspoon fresh thyme

1 teaspoon minced fresh rosemary

1 tablespoon minced shallot

½ cup extra-virgin olive oil

2 tablespoons water

¼ teaspoon fine sea salt

Freshly ground black pepper

1   In a high-speed blender, combine all of the ingredients and blend until the oil is emulsified. Taste and adjust any seasoning. Store in an airtight container in the refrigerator for up to 1 week until ready to use. (It will thicken slightly when chilled.)

creamy herb dressing

MAKES A GENEROUS 1 CUP | $0.39 PER SERVING

DF EF GF NF NS SF

½ cup raw tahini
(see Note)

½ cup water

3 tablespoons freshly
squeezed lemon juice

1 teaspoon raw apple
cider vinegar

1 clove garlic

½ teaspoon fine
sea salt

1 teaspoon onion
powder

1 tablespoon minced
fresh chives

1 tablespoon minced
fresh dill

1 teaspoon Dijon
mustard

This oil-free dressing is a great alternative to traditional creamy dressings because it's allergy-friendly and loaded with calcium, thanks to the use of raw tahini, a paste made from raw sesame seeds. It's hard to beat the flavor of fresh herbs in this recipe, but feel free to replace them with dried herbs if they are easier to find. When using dried herbs, be sure to reduce the amount you use by two-thirds, as their flavor is much more concentrated than the fresh variety. In general, 1 teaspoon of dried herbs is equivalent to 1 tablespoon of fresh herbs. You can taste as you go. Keep this creamy dressing on hand all week long for an easy ranchlike salad or quick veggie dip.

1 In a blender or food processor, combine all of the ingredients and blend until smooth and creamy. (Depending on the thickness of your tahini, you may want to add an additional 1 to 2 tablespoons water to help make the dressing more pourable.) Taste and adjust any seasoning. Serve immediately, or allow the dressing to chill in the refrigerator until ready to use. It will thicken a bit when chilled, making a thick dressing or veggie dip, but you can easily thin it out with additional water or lemon juice, as desired. Store leftovers in the refrigerator for up to 1 week.

NOTE: Be sure to use raw tahini for this recipe, if possible. Raw tahini is very light in color and mild in flavor, unlike roasted tahini, which is runny and very bitter. If you can't find the raw version with no added oil in your local store, you can order it online or make your own by grinding hulled raw sesame seeds in a food processor until smooth. (I buy my hulled raw seeds on Amazon—make sure they are hulled, though, or you'll wind up with inedible results.)

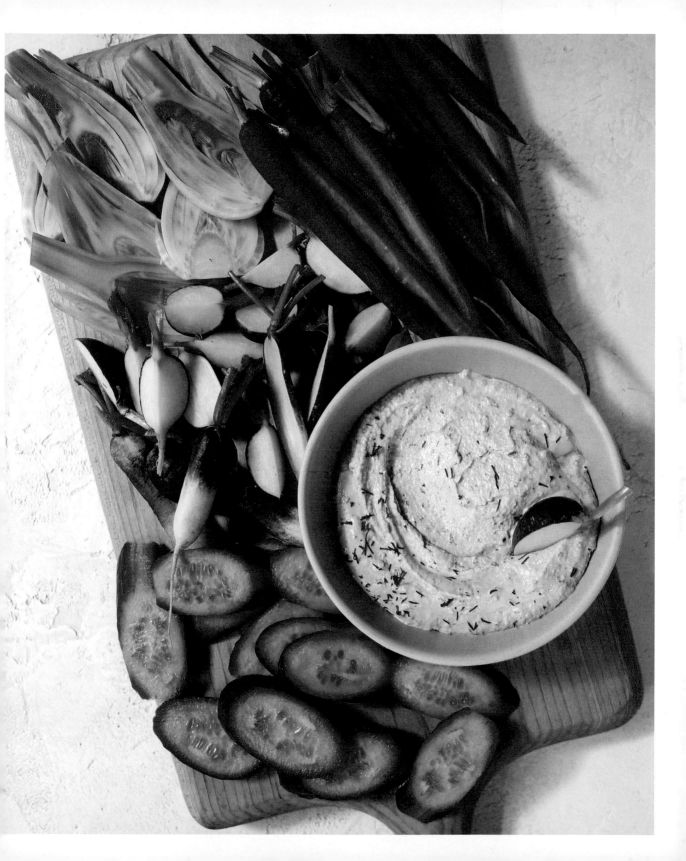

chopped salad
with creamy feta dressing

SERVES 4 | $2.99 PER SERVING

ANIMAL PROTEIN

DRESSING

4 ounces goat feta cheese, crumbled

2 tablespoons freshly squeezed lemon juice

¼ cup water

2 tablespoons olive oil

¼ teaspoon freshly ground black pepper

½ teaspoon dried oregano

1 clove garlic

1 tablespoon minced shallot

½ teaspoon raw honey

2 heads of romaine lettuce, chopped

1 large cucumber, chopped

1 cup cherry tomatoes, chopped

¼ red onion, chopped

1 red bell pepper, chopped

4 hard-boiled eggs, sliced

Freshly ground black pepper (optional)

For me, this recipe is really all about the dressing. It reminds me of my favorite dressing from a restaurant in Los Angeles called Granville. For years I tried to replicate their "lemon oregano" dressing without success, until I learned their secret recipe—they add a hefty dose of feta. No wonder it tastes so good. This version is remarkably close to theirs and is delicious over any number of juicy salad ingredients.

1 To prepare the dressing: In a high-speed blender, combine the cheese, lemon juice, water, olive oil, pepper, oregano, garlic, shallot, and honey. Blend until the oil is emulsified. Set aside to let the flavors meld while you prepare the salad.

2 In a large serving bowl, arrange the lettuce, cucumber, tomatoes, onion, bell pepper, and eggs. Pour the dressing over the top and toss to coat well. Serve immediately with additional freshly ground black pepper.

NOTE: This dressing is best used the day it's made since the garlic can become overpowering after sitting in the refrigerator overnight. If you want to prepare this dressing ahead of time, replace the fresh garlic with ¼ teaspoon garlic powder or blend in the garlic the day you plan to serve it.

carrot raisin slaw

SERVES 4 | $1.03 PER SERVING

30-MINUTE RECIPE
KID-FRIENDLY

This refreshing salad is a delicious alternative to creamy coleslaw and is almost always a hit with kids! Keep in mind that flavors tend to mellow the longer any salad sits, so if you plan on making this in advance, you might need to add a bit more lemon juice, salt, or honey right before serving to brighten it up. Luckily, this recipe is easy to taste as you go.

NUT/SEED/DRIED FRUIT

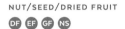

1   In a large bowl, whisk together the lemon juice, olive oil, honey, salt, and a few grinds of pepper. Add the carrots, green onions, parsley, raisins, and pecans and toss well to coat.

2   Cover and refrigerate for at least 15 minutes before serving to let the flavors meld. Store leftovers in an airtight container in the refrigerator for up to 4 days.

2 tablespoons freshly squeezed lemon juice

2 tablespoons extra-virgin olive oil

1 tablespoon raw honey

¼ teaspoon fine sea salt

Freshly ground black pepper

1 pound carrots, shredded

2 green onions, white and light green parts, thinly sliced

¼ cup chopped fresh Italian parsley

½ cup raisins

½ cup crushed pecans

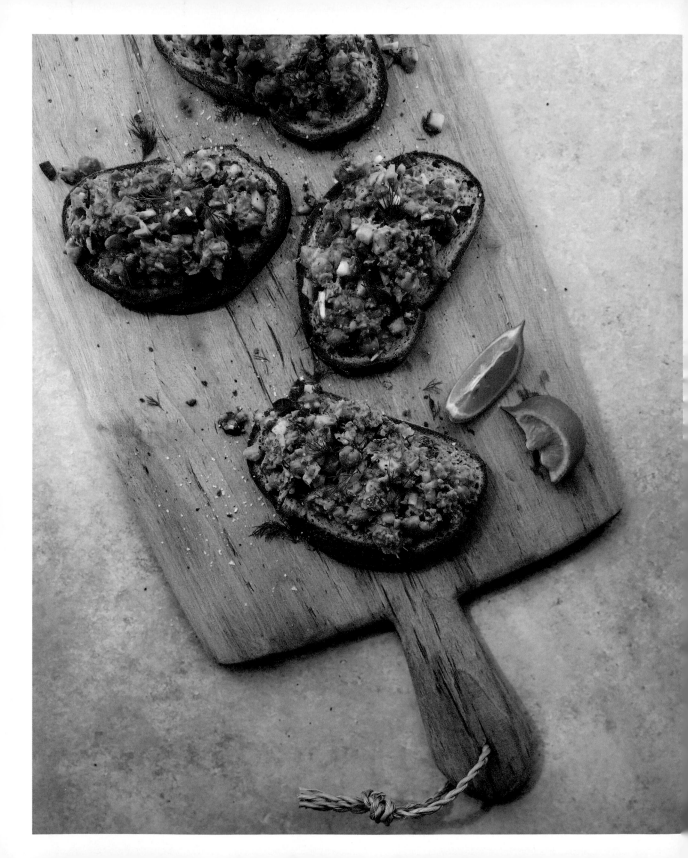

chickpea & avocado "egg" salad

SERVES 2 TO 4 | $1.58 TO $3.16 PER SERVING

30-MINUTE RECIPE

This recipe tastes ridiculously similar to traditional egg salad, but there's nothing traditional about it. A combination of chickpeas and creamy avocado gives this dish an egglike texture, and when paired with mustard, dill, and some crunchy veggies, it becomes a satisfying salad or sandwich filling that you'll crave. For a properly combined meal, serve this salad in lettuce cups, over a bed of greens, or between two slices of your favorite whole-grain bread.

1 In a large bowl, combine the chickpeas and avocado and roughly mash them together with a fork.

2 Add the mustard, lemon juice, salt, onion, bell pepper, cucumber, and dill to the bowl and then stir well to combine. Taste and adjust the seasonings before serving. Store leftovers in an airtight container in the refrigerator for up to 2 days, but keep in mind that it will brown slightly the longer it sits. Stir well again before serving.

STARCH

(DF) (EF) (GF) (NF) (SF) (NS) (V)

1½ cups cooked chickpeas (see page 78) or 1 (15-ounce) can, rinsed and drained well

1 ripe Hass avocado

2 teaspoons Dijon mustard

1 tablespoon freshly squeezed lemon juice

½ teaspoon fine sea salt

¼ cup diced red onion

¼ cup diced red bell pepper

½ cup diced cucumber

2 tablespoons minced fresh dill

roasted beet & goat cheese salad

SERVES 4 | $0.89 PER SERVING

ANIMAL PROTEIN

4 whole beets, red
or yellow

2 tablespoons raw
apple cider vinegar

2 tablespoons extra-
virgin olive oil

1 tablespoon raw honey

1 teaspoon Dijon
mustard

1 small shallot, chopped

Fine sea salt and
freshly ground black
pepper

3 cups mixed greens

3 ounces chèvre (soft
goat cheese), crumbled

This is my go-to salad when I'm looking to impress my dinner guests. Unlike other cooking methods, roasting brings out a natural sweetness in beets that pairs perfectly with tangy goat cheese and a quick shallot dressing. This salad is a breeze to put together, but it does require up to an hour of roasting time—feel free to roast the beets up to 4 days in advance.

1   Preheat the oven to 400°F. Trim the greens off the beets and arrange the beets in a small oven-safe pot, covered with a lid. (I use my 3.5-quart Dutch oven to avoid using aluminum foil as a cover.) Place in the oven and roast until a knife is easily inserted into the centers, 45 to 60 minutes, depending on the size of the beets. Allow the beets to cool before removing the skins—they should slip off easily (wear gloves to avoid staining your hands). Once peeled, chop the beets into chunks and set aside.

2   In a large bowl, combine the vinegar, olive oil, honey, mustard, and shallot; season with salt and pepper; and whisk well to combine. Add the beets and toss them in the dressing to coat.

3   Arrange the mixed greens on a large serving dish and spoon the dressed beets over the top. Drizzle any remaining dressing over the greens. Sprinkle with goat cheese and serve. (The dressing will be magenta if you use red beets, which is why you will want to add the goat cheese last—so it stays white on top.) Store leftovers in an airtight container in the refrigerator for up to 3 days.

MAKE IT AHEAD: You can let the roasted beets marinate in this dressing for up to 3 days in advance when stored in an airtight container in the refrigerator. To serve, simply spoon the dressed beets over fresh mixed greens and top with goat cheese for a quick and easy salad.

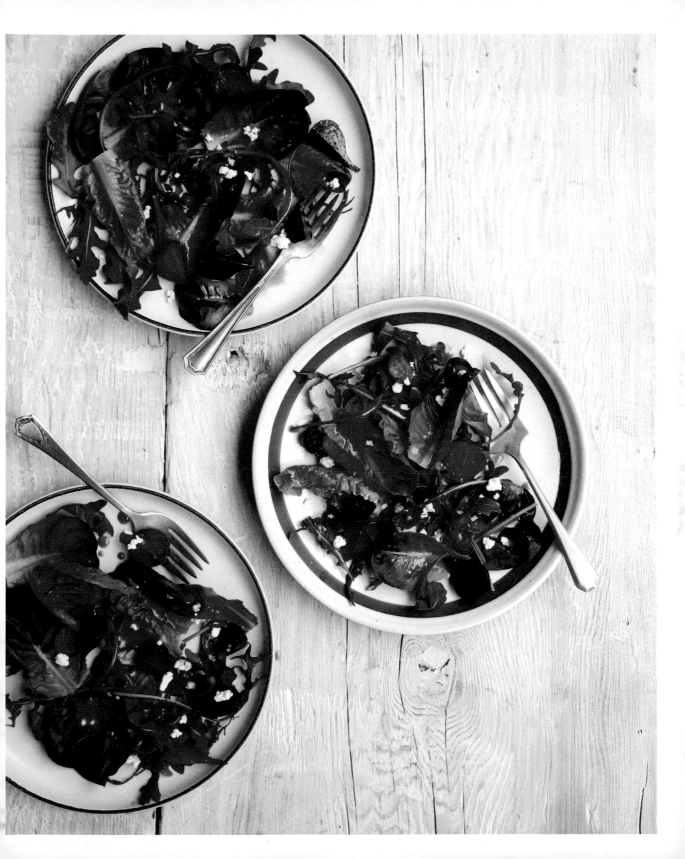

pizza salad

SERVES 2 TO 4 | $1.59 TO $3.18 PER SERVING

ANIMAL PROTEIN

DRESSING

2 sun-dried tomato halves, soaked in water for 15 minutes (see Note)

2 tablespoons raw apple cider vinegar

¼ cup extra-virgin olive oil

¼ cup water

1 clove garlic

¼ teaspoon fine sea salt

½ teaspoon dried oregano

⅛ teaspoon freshly ground black pepper

1 teaspoon maple syrup

2 heads of romaine lettuce, chopped

1 green bell pepper, chopped

1 cup cherry tomatoes, sliced in half

½ cup pitted black olives, sliced in half

½ cup diced red onion

½ cup shredded goat cheddar, mozzarella, or crumbled feta

If you're like me, you might always be looking for new ways to enjoy your favorite pizza ingredients without eating greasy pizza every single night. This salad (pictured on page iv, opposite the dedication) is my new favorite way to do just that. It features a mouthwatering sun-dried tomato dressing that is loaded with pizzalike flavor, poured over a bed of greens with the rest of my favorite pizza toppings, like green bell peppers, cheese, and occasionally even some nitrate-free pepperoni. (Because with this approach to detox, it's what you do *most* of the time that counts.) Feel free to use your favorite pizza toppings on this salad, as if it were your own personal pan pizza.

1   To prepare the dressing: In a high-speed blender, combine the tomatoes, vinegar, olive oil, water, garlic, salt, oregano, pepper, and maple syrup and blend until completely smooth. Taste and adjust any seasoning and set it aside.

2   In a large bowl, combine the lettuce, bell pepper, tomatoes, olives, onion, and cheese, and pour the dressing over the top. Toss well to coat. Serve immediately. This salad will wilt rather quickly after it's dressed, so if you want to save a portion for later, store the salad and dressing separately in airtight containers in the refrigerator for up to 3 days.

NOTE: I prefer to use sun-dried tomatoes that are not packed in oil, which is why they need to be soaked to help them soften. If you use the oil-packed version instead, soaking isn't necessary, although I would rinse them well to remove any excess oil.

creamy kale salad

SERVES 4 | $1.30 PER SERVING

30-MINUTE RECIPE
KID-FRIENDLY

This oil-free salad is a breeze to throw together and makes a satisfying main course or side dish. When you mix the dressing directly into the bottom of a large serving bowl and pile the greens on top, you'll dirty only one dish and speed the prep time. Kale is a nutritional powerhouse loaded with folate, a B vitamin key for brain development, as well as vitamins A, C, and K, and it packs 3 grams of protein per cup. Since it's such a sturdy green, any leftover salad can be packed for an easy lunch the next day!

NUT/SEED/DRIED FRUIT

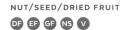

1. In a large bowl, combine the tahini, lemon juice, garlic, maple syrup, and salt. Season with pepper and add the water as needed to thin. Add the kale and toss with your hands to massage the dressing in. (Prepare to get your hands dirty!) The leaves will wilt slightly, making them more tender and helping to absorb the flavor of the dressing.

2. Toss in the carrots, raisins, and almonds and serve immediately or chill until ready to serve. Store leftovers in an airtight container in the refrigerator for up to 48 hours (before it becomes too soggy).

⅓ cup raw tahini

¼ cup freshly squeezed lemon juice

1 clove garlic, minced

2 teaspoons maple syrup

¼ teaspoon fine sea salt

Freshly ground black pepper

1 to 2 tablespoons water

1 pound lacinato kale, stems removed and leaves coarsely chopped

2 carrots, shredded

½ cup raisins

½ cup slivered almonds

mediterranean quinoa salad

SERVES 6 | $1.86 PER SERVING

STARCH

(DF) (EF) (GF) (NF) (SF) (NS) (V)

2 cups quinoa, rinsed
and drained

4 cups water

½ cup freshly squeezed
lemon juice

¼ cup extra-virgin
olive oil

2 teaspoons fine
sea salt

Freshly ground black
pepper

1 cup minced green
onions, white and
green parts

½ red onion, chopped

1 cup loosely packed
chopped fresh dill

1 cup loosely packed
chopped fresh flat-leaf
parsley

1 cucumber, chopped

1 large red bell pepper,
chopped

10 to 15 olives, chopped
(such as Castelvetrano)

Despite its reputation as a supergrain, quinoa is not technically a grain—
it's a seed (see Note). This particular seed happens to be a complete protein,
containing all nine essential amino acids, and is also a great source of iron,
magnesium, vitamin B$_2$, and manganese, all of which are necessary for healthy
brain function. Combined with an assortment of fresh herbs, olive oil, and
crunchy chopped vegetables, this salad is bursting with flavor and will make a
welcome addition to any party or gathering. The leftovers also make an easy
packed lunch for the week.

---

1   In a saucepan, combine the quinoa and water and bring to a boil. Cover and
    lower the heat, cooking until the quinoa has absorbed all of the water, about
    15 minutes. Fluff with a fork and allow to cool.

2   In a large bowl, whisk together the lemon juice, olive oil, salt, and a few
    grinds of pepper. Add the cooked quinoa and toss in the dressing to coat
    well. Add the green onion, red onion, dill, parsley, cucumber, bell pepper,
    and olives, and toss well to combine. Allow the mixture to marinate in the
    refrigerator for 1 hour before serving. This salad may be served cold or at
    room temperature. Store leftovers in an airtight container in the refrigerator
    for up to 4 days.

NOTE: Although quinoa is technically a seed, its grainlike quality places it in the
starch category for food combining. The same goes for other grainlike seeds, such
as amaranth, millet, and buckwheat. However, feel free to experiment to see how
this pseudograin best digests for you.

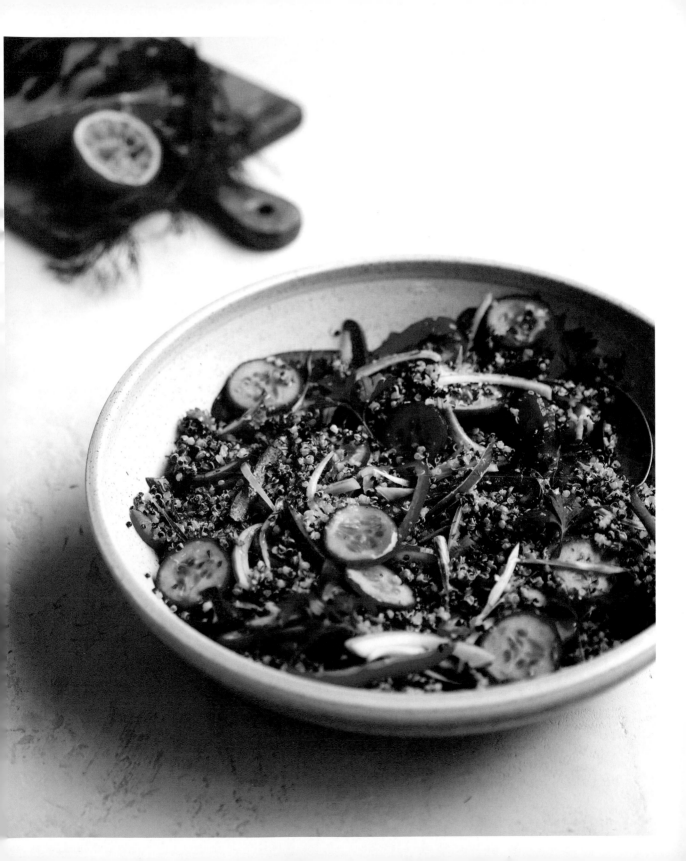

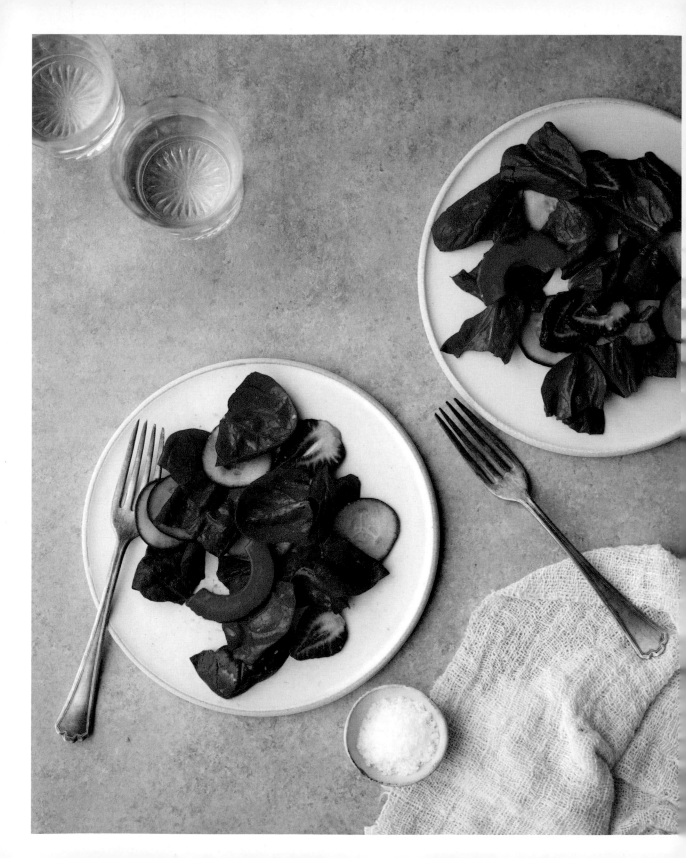

summer strawberry spinach salad

SERVES 4 | $2.44 PER SERVING

Fresh fruit doesn't make an appearance too often in food-combining recipes because it is digested so quickly, but this salad is an exception because strawberries pair perfectly with leafy greens and other fruits, like creamy avocado and crunchy cucumbers. This salad is best served during the summer months, when fresh strawberries are at their peak of sweetness.

1 To prepare the dressing: In a high-speed blender, combine the vinegar, olive oil, shallot, water, maple syrup, mustard, and garlic and blend until smooth and the oil is emulsified. Set aside.

2 In a large bowl, arrange the spinach, strawberries, avocado, and cucumber. Pour the dressing over the top and toss to coat. (You don't have to use all of the dressing if you don't want to—taste it as you go.) Serve immediately. This salad will wilt rather quickly after it's dressed, so if you want to save a portion for later, store the salad and dressing separately in airtight containers in the refrigerator for up to 3 days.

NOTE: If food combining isn't a concern for you, this salad is extra tasty with the addition of sprinkled feta cheese.

FRESH FRUIT

DRESSING

2 tablespoons raw apple cider vinegar

¼ cup extra-virgin olive oil

1 tablespoon minced shallot

1 tablespoon water

1½ tablespoons maple syrup

1 teaspoon Dijon mustard

1 clove garlic

6 cups fresh baby spinach

1 pint strawberries, sliced

1 ripe Hass avocado, sliced

1 cucumber, quartered and cut into ¼-inch chunks

crunchy thai salad
with creamy "peanut" dressing

SERVES 4 | $1.63 PER SERVING

NUT/SEED/DRIED FRUIT

DF EF GF NF

DRESSING

¼ cup sunflower
seed butter

1 tablespoon raw
apple cider vinegar

2 tablespoons extra-
virgin olive oil

2 tablespoons freshly
squeezed lemon juice

1 tablespoon tamari
(gluten-free soy sauce)

3 tablespoons raw
honey

1 clove garlic, minced

1-inch knob of fresh
ginger, peeled and
chopped

¼ teaspoon fine
sea salt

¼ teaspoon crushed r
ed pepper flakes

¼ cup water, or more
to thin

2 heads of romaine
lettuce, shredded

½ head of cabbage,
shredded, or
1 (12-ounce) bag

3 carrots, shredded

1 red bell pepper,
chopped

½ cup hulled sunflower
seeds

One of the keys to enjoying salads on a regular basis is finding a salad dressing that you love—and this one is always a huge hit with everyone. It reminds me of the creamy peanut dressings served at Thai restaurants, but it's made with sunflower seed butter as an allergy-friendly alternative. Paired with crunchy cabbage, juicy romaine, and sweet shredded carrots, this salad makes a filling entrée on its own, and any leftover dressing makes a great veggie dip that you can store in the refrigerator as a quick snack.

1   To prepare the dressing: In a high-speed blender, combine the seed butter, vinegar, olive oil, lemon juice, tamari, honey, garlic, ginger, salt, red pepper flakes, and water and blend until completely smooth. Set aside.

2   In a large bowl, combine the lettuce, cabbage, carrots, bell pepper, and sunflower seeds. Pour the dressing over the top and toss well to coat. Serve immediately. This salad will wilt rather quickly after it's dressed, so if you want to save a portion for later, store the salad and dressing separately in airtight containers in the refrigerator for up to 3 days.

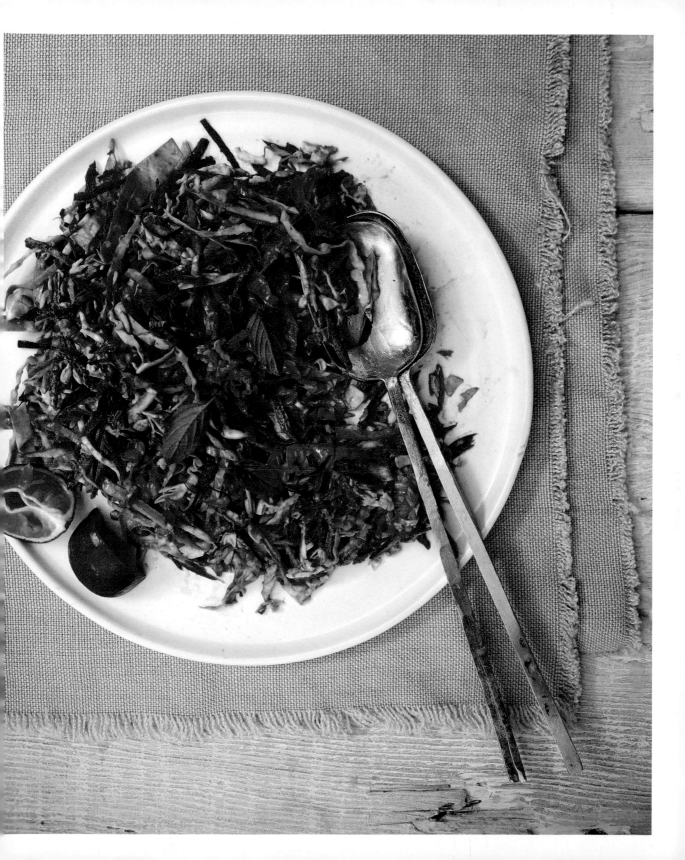

shredded brussels sprout salad

SERVES 2 TO 4 | $1.24 TO $2.47 PER SERVING

ANIMAL PROTEIN

EF GF NF NS SF

2 tablespoons extra-virgin olive oil

2 tablespoons raw apple cider vinegar

2 teaspoons Dijon mustard

¼ teaspoon fine sea salt

Freshly ground black pepper

1 pound brussels sprouts, shredded (see Note)

1 red bell pepper, chopped

½ cup diced red onion

¼ cup grated Pecorino Romano cheese

This salad reminds me of a fresh and crunchy Greek salad but with a refreshing twist, since it uses brussels sprouts instead of romaine lettuce. Brussels sprouts are an excellent source of vitamin C and contain compounds called glucosinolates that may help reduce cancer risk,[2] so this salad is an excellent way to sneak more of these healthy nutrients into your diet. When you shred the brussels sprouts finely enough, no one can even tell that they're not eating lettuce. This salad is durable enough to sit in the dressing overnight, so leftovers make an easy packed lunch the next day, too.

1   In a large bowl, combine the olive oil, vinegar, mustard, and salt; season with pepper; and whisk to combine. Add the brussels sprouts, bell pepper, and onion and toss well to coat. Stir in the cheese and, for the best flavor, allow the salad to marinate for at least 15 minutes before serving. If you plan on making this salad more than an hour in advance, be sure to taste it before serving. Flavors tend to mellow as they sit, so you may need to add a touch more vinegar to the bowl to brighten it up.

NOTE: You can use a food processor to quickly shred the brussels sprouts, but I prefer to use a good knife and cutting board to avoid washing an extra appliance. Either way works.

avocado caesar salad

SERVES 2 TO 4 | $1.84 TO $3.68 PER SERVING

15-MINUTE PREP

Caesar salads are always a crowd-pleaser, but since most of them are loaded with cheese and excess oil, they're not always the healthiest choice. Luckily, this salad is almost as satisfying as the original, getting its creaminess from heart-healthy avocado and a "cheesy" flavor from nutritional yeast. With a hefty serving of garlic, a signature ingredient in any Caesar dressing, this salad may not be the best option to serve on a first date, but it certainly will give your immune system a boost! Top this salad with Crispy Garlic Chickpeas (page 115) for a protein-rich crouton.

1 To prepare the dressing: In a high-speed blender, combine the avocado, garlic, lemon juice, vinegar, water, mustard, salt, and nutritional yeast and blend until completely smooth. Adjust seasoning to taste, adding up to 2 more cloves of garlic.

2 Place the lettuce in a large bowl, pour in the dressing, and toss well to coat. Serve immediately. The lettuce will wilt quickly after it's dressed, so if you want to save a portion for later, store the lettuce and dressing separately in airtight containers in the refrigerator for up to 3 days.

STARCH

(DF) (EF) (GF) (NF) (SF) (NS) (V)

DRESSING

½ cup mashed ripe Hass avocado

3 to 5 cloves garlic, minced

2 tablespoons freshly squeezed lemon juice

1 teaspoon raw apple cider vinegar

¾ cup water

1 teaspoon Dijon mustard

½ teaspoon fine sea salt

2 tablespoons nutritional yeast

3 heads romaine lettuce, chopped

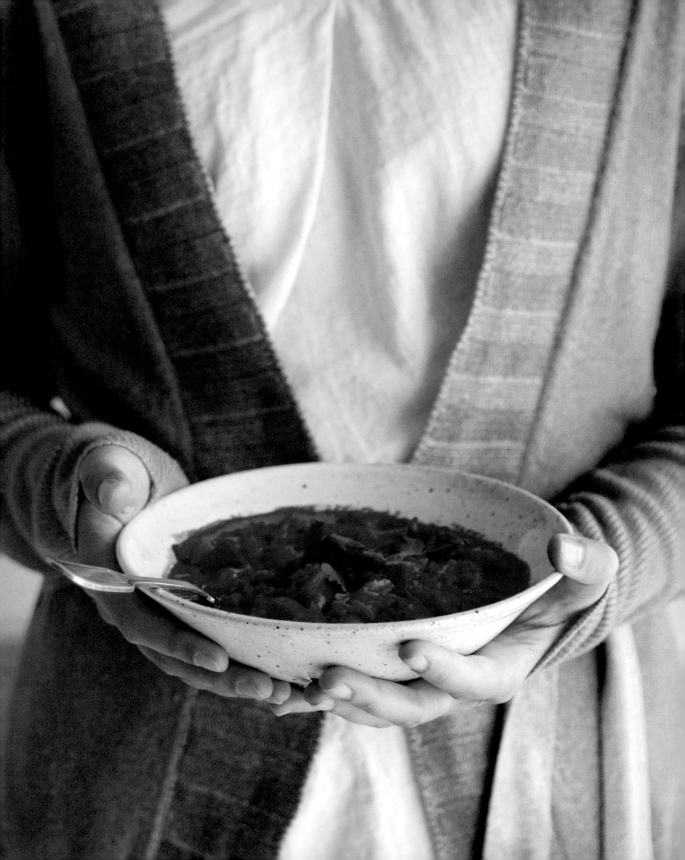

4 SOUPS & SIDES

tuscan bean soup

SERVES 4 | $2.26 PER SERVING

STARCH

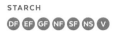

1 tablespoon
coconut oil

1 yellow onion, chopped

3 carrots, chopped

4 celery stalks, chopped

3 cloves garlic, minced

1 teaspoon minced
fresh thyme

1 teaspoon minced
fresh rosemary

¼ teaspoon red pepper
flakes

3 tomatoes, chopped

1 zucchini, quartered
and sliced into ½-inch
pieces

3 to 4 cups water

3 cups cooked
cannellini beans (see
page 78) or 2 (15-ounce)
cans, rinsed and
drained

Fine sea salt

3 cups lacinato
kale, ribs removed
and leaves coarsely
chopped

Freshly ground black
pepper

This is one of my family's favorite soups. The white beans provide an unbelievably creamy texture, along with a hearty serving of fiber and protein, and when paired with aromatic herbs like rosemary and thyme, you get an ultra-comforting dish that can be served as a main course along with a leafy green salad. Although the recipe calls for cannellini beans, feel free to use any other white bean easily available to you, such as great Northern or navy beans, for similar results.

1   In a large Dutch oven, melt the coconut oil over medium heat and sauté the onion, carrots, and celery until tender. Add the garlic, thyme, rosemary, and red pepper flakes and sauté for another minute, just until fragrant. Add the tomatoes and zucchini and sauté for 5 minutes to soften them.

2   Add 3 cups of the water along with the beans and 1 teaspoon salt and bring the soup to a boil. Lower the heat and stir in the kale, then cover and simmer for 15 minutes.

3   Season with black pepper and use an immersion blender to puree the soup a bit—leaving some texture but adding a creaminess to the overall base. If the soup is too thick, add some of the remaining 1 cup water and then season with additional salt. Serve warm. Store leftovers in an airtight container in the refrigerator for up to 4 days, or in the freezer for up to 3 months.

MAKE IT AHEAD: Use the Freezer or Slow/Pressure Cooker Method on page 15.

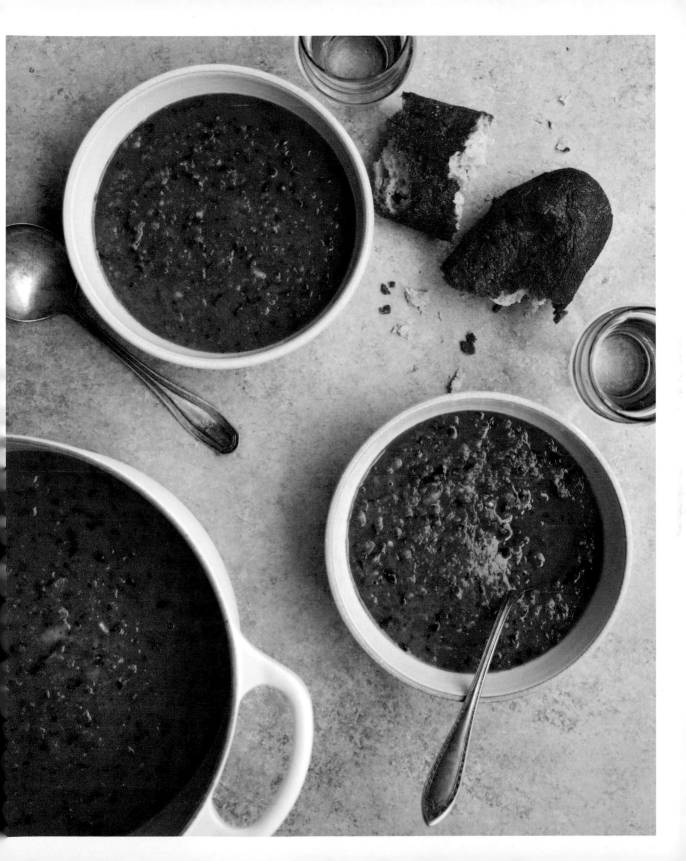

Cooking Beans from Scratch

While canned beans are convenient, dried beans are a more affordable alternative with very little hands-on time required. To prepare, soak the beans in a large container of water, covered and refrigerated, for about 8 hours. Use 5 cups of water for every 1 cup of dried beans, since they will expand as they soak. (This helps remove the starch that can cause gas and bloating.) Drain and rinse the soaked beans with fresh water before cooking. In a large pot, cover the beans with fresh water and bring to a boil, then lower the heat and simmer until the beans are tender, 1 to 2 hours depending on the type of bean; add more water periodically to keep the beans covered. Use a fork to mash a bean against the side of the pot periodically to check for tenderness. When they are tender, drain the cooked beans and use them in any recipe you like. After they are drained, cooked beans can be stored in an airtight container in the refrigerator for up to 4 days or in the freezer for up to 6 months.

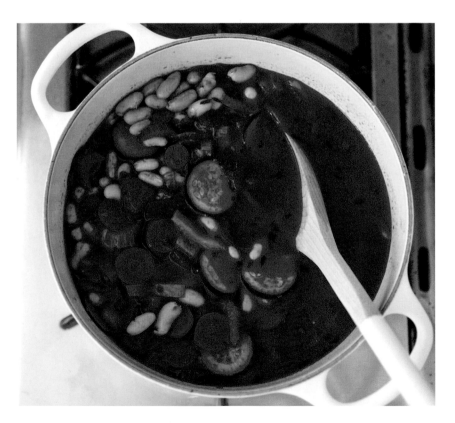

cauliflower & leek soup

SERVES 4 TO 6 | $1.17 TO $1.75 PER SERVING

This recipe reminds me of a lighter version of baked potato soup, and because it's entirely vegetable-based, you are welcome to load it up any way you like. A few of my family members like to add a sprinkle of cheese and crisp bacon over the top, but just a sprinkling of fresh chives is all the garnish you need with this flavorful and creamy soup. This simple recipe is surprisingly delicious and is loaded with antioxidants and phytonutrients, which may help protect your cells from exposure to everyday pollutants and stress.

NEUTRAL

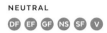

1 tablespoon coconut oil

2 celery stalks, chopped

2 cloves garlic, minced

3 leeks, white and light green parts, thinly sliced (see Note, page 45)

1 head of cauliflower, cut into florets

4 cups water

2 teaspoons fine sea salt

Freshly ground black pepper

½ cup almond milk or additional water, to thin

Chopped fresh chives, for garnish

1   In a large pot, melt the coconut oil over medium heat and sauté the celery, garlic, and leeks until tender, about 5 minutes. Feel free to use a splash of water during the sauté process to prevent sticking.

2   Add the cauliflower, water, salt, and pepper and bring to a boil. Cover and lower the heat to a simmer, cooking until the cauliflower is tender, 15 to 20 minutes. The cauliflower should be easily pierced with a fork when done.

3   Use an immersion blender to blend the soup directly in the pot or transfer the soup in batches to a traditional blender to process until smooth. (Be sure to leave the vent in your blender lid open to prevent the steam pressure from building up—it could blow the lid off your blender and cause burns. Instead, loosely cover the vent with a thin dish towel to prevent splattering.)

4   Return the soup to the pot and stir in the almond milk until a creamy texture is achieved and adjust any seasoning as needed. Serve warm with a garnish of fresh chives. Store leftovers in an airtight container in the refrigerator for up to 4 days, or in the freezer for up to 3 months.

MAKE IT AHEAD: Use the Freezer or Slow/Pressure Cooker Method on page 15.

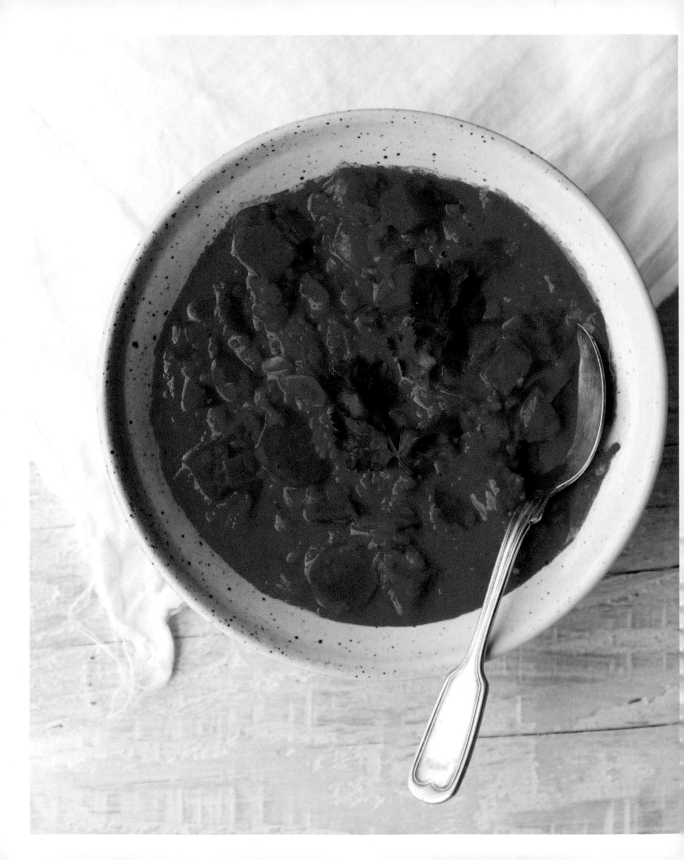

mock mulligatawny stew

SERVES 4 | $1.04 PER SERVING

If you haven't tried mulligatawny soup before, you don't know what you're missing. Despite its rather intimidating name, this soup was a huge hit at a restaurant where I used to work because its flavor and texture was so satisfying—a complete meal in a bowl. The traditional version is made with chicken, heavy cream, rice, and apples that can be a bit of a digestive disaster. I've simplified this vegetarian version while still packing in the sweet and spicy flavor and an extra dose of protein-rich lentils.

STARCH

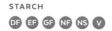

1 tablespoon
coconut oil

1 yellow onion, chopped

3 carrots, chopped

3 celery stalks, chopped

1 clove garlic, minced

1 tablespoon minced
fresh ginger

4 teaspoons
curry powder

5 cups water

1 pound unpeeled
sweet potatoes,
chopped

1 cup dried red lentils

Fine sea salt

½ cup full-fat
coconut milk

1 tablespoon freshly
squeezed lemon juice

1 to 2 tablespoons
maple syrup

Freshly ground black
pepper (optional)

1   In a large pot, melt the coconut oil over medium heat and sauté the onion, carrots, and celery until they start to get soft, about 5 minutes. Add the garlic, ginger, and curry powder and sauté until fragrant, about 1 minute.

2   Add the water, sweet potatoes, lentils, and 2 teaspoons salt and raise the heat to bring the mixture to a boil. Cover and lower the heat to a simmer, cooking until the lentils and potatoes are tender, 15 to 18 minutes.

3   Stir in the coconut milk and lemon juice, and sweeten with the maple syrup to taste. Season with salt (I usually add another ½ teaspoon) and pepper, if desired. Serve warm. Store leftovers in an airtight container in the refrigerator for up to 4 days, or in the freezer for up to 3 months.

MAKE IT AHEAD: Use the Freezer or Slow/Pressure Cooker Method on page 14.

creamy mushroom soup

SERVES 4 TO 6 | $0.82 TO $1.23 PER SERVING

STARCH

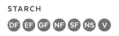

1 tablespoon coconut oil

1 small yellow onion,
chopped

2 cloves garlic, minced

1 pound baby bella
mushrooms, sliced

1 (8-ounce) Yukon gold
potato, cut into 1-inch
chunks

1½ teaspoons fine
sea salt

¼ cup coarsely chopped
fresh basil

4 to 5 cups water

1 cup nondairy milk
(optional)

1 teaspoon freshly
squeezed lemon juice

Freshly ground black
pepper

I developed this recipe for a close friend who is mildly obsessed with the creamy vegan mushroom soup served at Boma, a restaurant at the Walt Disney World Resort. This copycat version is easy to make at home, and, as an added perk, you'll be getting a healthy dose of selenium, which helps support the immune system, as well as niacin, which helps with carbohydrate, protein, and fat metabolism. Any leftover soup also makes a delicious sauce over pasta or as a gravy over mashed potatoes.

1   In a large pot, melt the coconut oil over medium heat, and sauté the onion until it begins to soften, about 5 minutes. Add the garlic and mushrooms and sauté until very tender and the mushrooms have released most of their moisture, about 10 minutes more.

2   Add the potato, salt, basil, and 4 cups of the water and bring the mixture to a boil. Once boiling, lower the heat to a simmer, then cover and cook until the potatoes are fork-tender, about 15 minutes.

3   Transfer the soup in batches to a traditional blender to process until creamy. (Be sure to leave the vent in your blender open to prevent the steam pressure from building up—it could blow the lid off your blender and cause burns. Instead, loosely cover the vent with a thin dish towel to prevent splattering.) You can blend all of the soup into a silky-smooth texture or reserve some of the sautéed mushrooms for some added texture in the final soup.

4   Return the soup to the pot. Add the remaining 1 cup water or the nondairy milk to give the soup a creamier and silkier texture, along with the lemon juice, and adjust the seasonings. Serve the soup piping hot, garnished with pepper. Store leftovers in an airtight container in the refrigerator for up to 4 days, or in the freezer for up to 3 months.

MAKE IT AHEAD: Use the Freezer or Slow/Pressure Cooker Method on page 15.

mexican quinoa stew

SERVES 4 TO 6 | $0.97 TO $1.46 PER SERVING

This hearty stew is a lighter vegetarian version of my family's favorite chicken tortilla soup. Instead of using tortillas, this soup is thickened with protein-rich quinoa and black beans for a filling alternative. Although using an immersion blender to partially blend this soup is optional, I highly recommend it, since it makes the texture much more satisfying and more like traditional tortilla soup. Seasoned with cumin, which is known for aiding digestion and improving immunity, this soup is perfect for any time you need a warm, comforting, and healthful meal.

STARCH

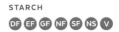

1 teaspoon coconut oil

1 yellow onion, chopped

2 celery stalks, chopped

3 carrots, chopped

4 cloves garlic, minced

2 jalapeño chiles, seeded and chopped

3½ cups water

1 (28-ounce) box or jar chopped tomatoes

1½ cups cooked black beans (see page 78) or 1 (15-ounce) can, rinsed and drained

1½ teaspoons ground cumin

2 teaspoons fine sea salt

½ cup quinoa

¼ cup chopped fresh cilantro

⅛ teaspoon cayenne pepper (optional)

Freshly ground black pepper

1   In a large pot, melt the coconut oil over medium heat, and sauté the onion, celery, carrots, garlic, and jalapeños until tender, about 8 minutes.

2   Add the water, tomatoes, beans, cumin, salt, quinoa, cilantro, and cayenne; season with pepper; and bring the soup to a boil.

3   Once boiling, lower the heat, cover the pot, and let simmer until the quinoa is tender, about 15 minutes. Once the quinoa is tender, adjust any seasonings. You can serve the soup right away or use an immersion blender to puree a bit of the soup—this helps it thicken while still leaving some texture. Store leftovers in an airtight container in the refrigerator for up to 4 days, or in the freezer for up to 3 months.

MAKE IT AHEAD: Use the Freezer or Slow/Pressure Cooker Method on page 15.

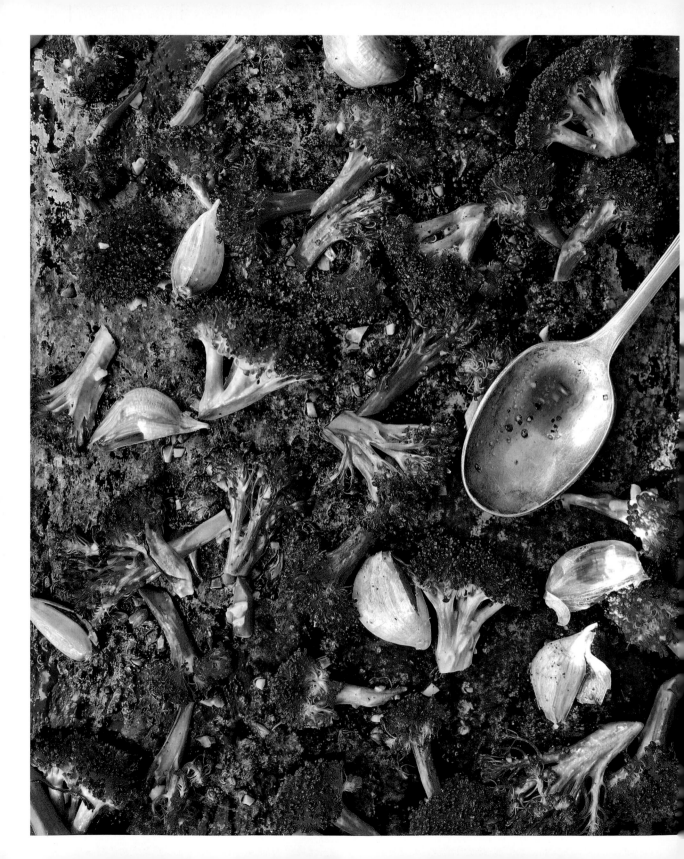

addictive garlic-roasted broccoli

SERVES 4 | $0.68 PER SERVING

Roasted broccoli is already a popular side dish, but this recipe takes it to the next level. The addition of lemon juice really brightens up the flavor, and when you add a sprinkling of grated cheese, no one will be able to turn it down. As it turns out, cooked broccoli aids in lowering cholesterol more effectively than eating it raw, and it contains a special combination of phytonutrients that support the body's natural detoxification process. While I wouldn't plan on having any leftovers, this roasted vegetable also makes a great salad topper for a future meal.

ANIMAL PROTEIN

1 Preheat the oven to 350°F.

2 In a large bowl, toss the broccoli with the coconut oil, lemon juice, and garlic and arrange in a single layer on a large baking sheet. Sprinkle generously with sea salt.

3 Bake for about 30 minutes, until the broccoli is lightly brown and fork-tender. Remove from the oven and sprinkle with the cheese. Toss well to coat and serve immediately. Store leftovers in an airtight container in the refrigerator for up to 3 days.

NOTE: To ensure quick and even roasting, be sure to slice each broccoli stem in half. The stems are usually the part that take the longest to cook, leaving the florets burned by the time the stems are fork-tender. Burnt vegetables can be a sign of acrylamide formation, a cancer-causing substance (see page 103), so you definitely don't want to eat burnt broccoli!

1 pound broccoli florets (see Note)

2 tablespoons coconut oil, melted

1 tablespoon freshly squeezed lemon juice

1 clove garlic, minced

Fine sea salt

3 to 4 tablespoons grated Pecorino Romano cheese (optional)

creamy cauliflower "potato" salad

SERVES 4 TO 6 | $0.88 TO XX PER SERVING

STARCH

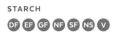

1 (2-pound) head of cauliflower, cut into florets

1 ripe Hass avocado

2 tablespoons Dijon mustard

1 teaspoon freshly squeezed lemon juice

¼ teaspoon fine sea salt

2 tablespoons minced shallot

2 tablespoons minced fresh dill

2 tablespoons minced fresh chives

1 cup diced cucumber

2 celery stalks, diced

This is one of my new favorite side dishes to share at a barbecue or picnic. It tastes like a cross between egg salad and potato salad, but it's made with lower-starch cauliflower instead of potatoes and is vegan to boot! Instead of using a store-bought vegan mayonnaise or cashew-based alternative, this dish gets its creaminess from an avocado, making it as quick and easy as possible. Because avocado does tend to brown quickly, it's best to make this salad the same day you plan to serve it, but you can cook and chill the cauliflower up to 2 days in advance to save on prep time.

1   Fill a large pot with 1 inch of water, fit it with a steamer basket, and add the cauliflower. Bring the water to a boil, then lower the heat to a simmer and cover the pot to let the cauliflower steam until tender but not mushy, about 10 minutes.

2   While the cauliflower is steaming, in a large bowl, combine the avocado, mustard, lemon juice, and salt and use a fork to mash the mixture together until relatively smooth. Add the shallot, dill, chives, cucumber, and celery and stir to combine.

3   Once the cauliflower is tender, drain well and add it to the avocado mixture. Stir well to combine and adjust any seasonings. Place the salad in the refrigerator to chill for 2 hours before serving, and taste again once chilled to make sure the flavors are to your liking. (You might want to add a little more mustard or lemon juice to brighten it up.)

NOTE: Not a fan of cauliflower? This recipe also works well with steamed Yukon gold potato chunks, which contain 45 percent of the recommended daily value for vitamin C. Or, for a slightly sweeter version, try using white sweet potatoes, which are also loaded with vitamins A and C.

soy-ginger green beans

SERVES 4 | $0.98 PER SERVING

15-MINUTE PREP

I'm always looking for new ways to prepare vegetables, and these green beans make the perfect side dish for a number of main entrées. They are flavorful without being overpowering, and they take about 10 minutes to cook from start to finish! Green beans are loaded with antioxidants like lutein and beta-carotene and provide a good source of silicon, which is a mineral important for bone health. Any leftover green beans would be delicious served over the Crunchy Thai Salad on page 70.

1   In a large, deep skillet, melt the coconut oil over medium heat and sauté the ginger and garlic for about 1 minute, just until fragrant. Add the green beans and sauté for 2 minutes, then add the water and partially cover the pot with a lid to let the beans cook until crisp-tender, about 4 minutes.

2   Remove the lid and add the tamari and maple syrup. Toss well to coat and stir until the liquid is dissolved, 1 to 2 minutes more. Remove from the heat and stir in the sesame oil. Serve warm.

NOTE: While sesame oil is high in antioxidants that offer some protective properties, its polyunsaturated fat content can make it less stable as a cooking oil. That is why I recommend turning off the heat before adding it at the end of this recipe, using it only for flavor. Store this oil in an airtight container in the refrigerator for best shelf life after opening.

NEUTRAL

1 tablespoon coconut oil

2 teaspoons minced fresh ginger

1 teaspoon minced garlic

1 pound fresh green beans, cut into 1-inch pieces

¼ cup water

1 tablespoon tamari (gluten-free soy sauce)

1 teaspoon maple syrup

½ teaspoon sesame oil (see Note)

cinnamon-glazed carrots

SERVES 4 | $0.50 PER SERVING

NEUTRAL

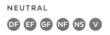

1 teaspoon coconut oil

1 pound baby carrots, sliced carrot coins, or halved large carrots

½ cup water

1 to 2 tablespoons maple syrup

1 teaspoon ground cinnamon

Pinch of fine sea salt

Eating vegetables is so important that it doesn't necessarily matter what you top them with if it helps your picky family members eat them more often. If you ask me, topping your veggies with a sprinkling of cheese or a little bit of natural sugar is far better than eating no veggies at all, and this quick side dish is an easy way to get started. The addition of cinnamon and naturally sweet maple syrup makes these carrots taste like dessert, plus they can be ready in just 15 minutes!

1   In a Dutch oven, melt the coconut oil over medium heat and sauté the carrots for 2 minutes. Add the water, which should start bubbling right away, and lower the heat to a simmer. Partially cover the pot and cook the carrots for about 10 minutes, until fork-tender. Check the pot periodically to make sure the water doesn't completely evaporate so the carrots don't burn.

2   Once the carrots are tender, raise the heat to cook off any excess water, then stir in the maple syrup, cinnamon, and salt. Adjust the seasonings. Serve warm. Leftovers can be stored in an airtight container in the refrigerator for up to 3 days.

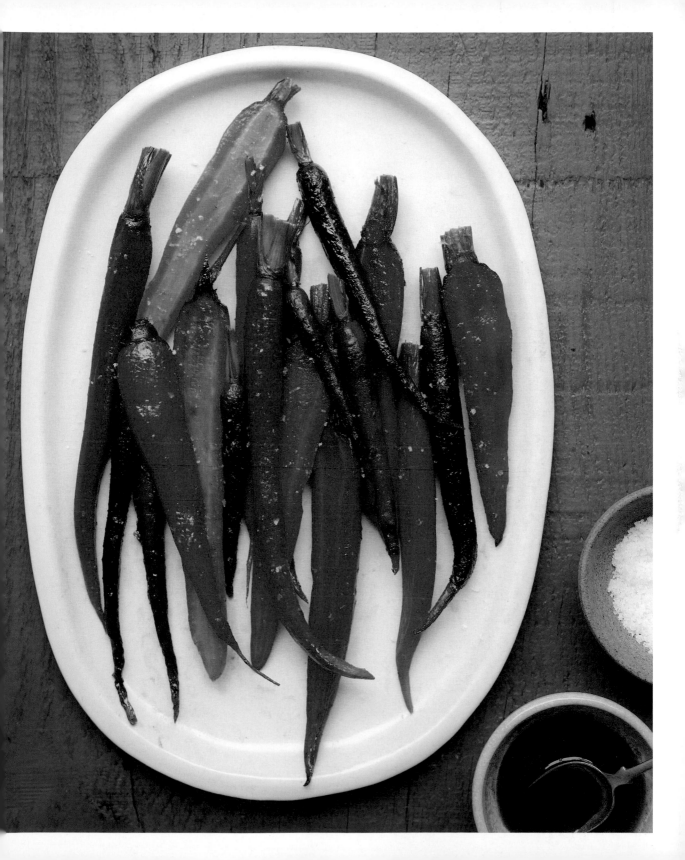

slow-cooker cinnamon applesauce

MAKES ABOUT 40 OUNCES | $0.47 PER SERVING

FRESH FRUIT

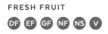

3 pounds red sweet apples, such as Jonathan or McIntosh

½ cup water

1 teaspoon ground cinnamon

Calling for only three ingredients, this recipe is just about as easy as it gets. What I love about making my own applesauce at home is that you have total control over the additives and preservatives, which I feel is especially important when feeding children. This applesauce is so naturally sweet, there's no need for any added sugar, anyway!

1   Peel and core the apples, cut them into large slices, and then place them in the bowl of a slow cooker along with the water and cinnamon. Stir once to combine, then cover and set to cook on low for 6 hours, or until the apples are very soft. (If you have an electric pressure cooker, cook on "high" for 10 minutes, and then let the pressure naturally release.)

2   Use a potato masher or an immersion blender to gently puree the applesauce directly in the pot, or you can transfer in batches to a traditional blender if you prefer. Be careful not to overblend because you don't want your applesauce to have the texture of baby food. (Unless, of course, you're making this for a baby!) Store the applesauce in an airtight container in the refrigerator for up to 10 days or in the freezer (in batches to extend shelf life) for up to 6 months.

NOTE: If you don't mind the texture of a smoother applesauce made in the blender, you can leave the peels of the apples on for more nutrition. The peels become very soft when baked and are easily pureed into the sauce when blended. Alternatively, you can use the fresh apple peels in your next smoothie to avoid wasting that nutrition.

FRUIT-FLAVORED VARIATIONS: If your kids are like mine, they might be drawn to the popular flavored-applesauce pouches on the market. I like to make my own fun variations at home by adding 1 pound of chopped frozen fruit to the recipe and omitting the cinnamon. My son's favorite additions are mango and peach.

quick bread & butter pickles

MAKES ONE 16-OUNCE JAR | $4 FOR THE WHOLE JAR

If you're like me, you might be too timid or time constrained to learn how to properly ferment a jar of homemade pickles, so this recipe is my quick and easy solution. You can enjoy these pickles as soon as they cool, so there's no need to wait weeks for them to be ready. Once you master this method, adjust the seasonings as you see fit to make your own perfect pickle.

NEUTRAL

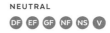

⅓ cup raw apple cider vinegar

½ cup water

¼ cup maple syrup

1 teaspoon fine sea salt

1 clove garlic, crushed

1 (8-ounce) cucumber, cut into ¼-inch slices

2 tablespoons chopped fresh dill

1 In a saucepan, combine the vinegar, water, maple syrup, salt, and garlic over high heat and bring the mixture to a boil. Once boiling, lower the heat and simmer for 5 minutes to let the flavors meld.

2 Arrange the cucumbers and fresh dill in a large bowl and pour the hot liquid over the top. Toss well to coat.

3 Transfer the pickles to a 16-ounce mason jar, making sure the liquid covers the cucumber slices (add a little water if you need to). Place the jar in the refrigerator to allow the pickles to cool. Once chilled, you can serve them right away, but the flavor gets even better the following day. Store the jar in the refrigerator for up to 1 month.

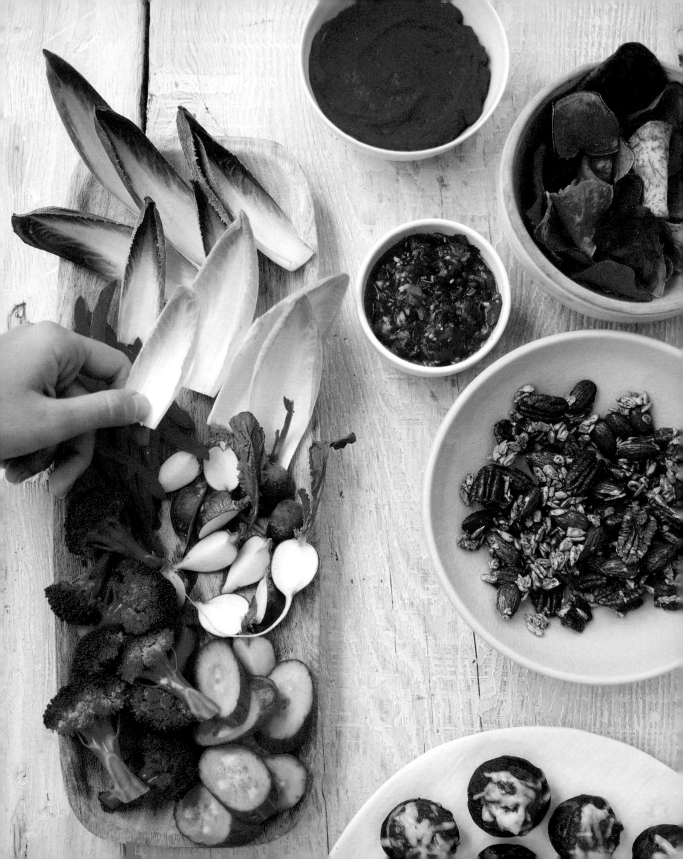

5 GAME-DAY APPETIZERS & SNACKS ON THE GO

savory sweet potato crackers

MAKES ABOUT 25 CRACKERS | $0.66 PER SERVING

STARCH

(DF) (EF) (GF) (NF) (SF) (NS) (V)

½ cup mashed
sweet potato

¾ cup gluten-free oat
flour (see page 189)

½ teaspoon fine
sea salt

1 teaspoon minced
fresh rosemary

¼ teaspoon
garlic powder

2 tablespoons
coconut oil, melted

These allergy-friendly crackers are a great alternative to the store-bought varieties that are loaded with refined flour and sodium. They pack a sneaky serving of sweet potato into each bite, which provides a good source of potassium and vitamin A while still satisfying that craving for something crunchy and savory. Serve them with your favorite dip or pack them as an easy snack on the go.

1   Preheat the oven to 350°F and line a large baking sheet with parchment paper. In a large mixing bowl, combine the sweet potato, flour, salt, rosemary, garlic powder, and coconut oil and stir well to create a uniform dough.

2   Transfer the dough to the prepared baking sheet and top it with another sheet of parchment paper. Use a rolling pin to roll the dough into a thin layer, about ⅛ inch thick. The thinner you roll the dough, the crispier your crackers will get, and the faster they will cook. Gently remove the top layer of parchment paper and use a pizza cutter to cut the crackers into 1-inch squares.

3   Bake for 15 minutes, then remove the baking sheet from the oven and use a spatula to flip each cracker for even baking (they should split apart easily where you cut them).

4   Return the pan to the oven to bake until the crackers are dry and crisp, about 15 minutes more. Be sure to watch the crackers closely toward the end of the baking time, since the edge pieces will cook faster than the center pieces, and the crackers won't taste as good if they turn dark brown. Remove any pieces by the edge of the pan when they are done and continue cooking the center crackers until they are all dry, checking on them every 3 to 5 minutes. Allow the crackers to cool completely for the crispiest results. Store in an airtight container at room temperature for up to 5 days.

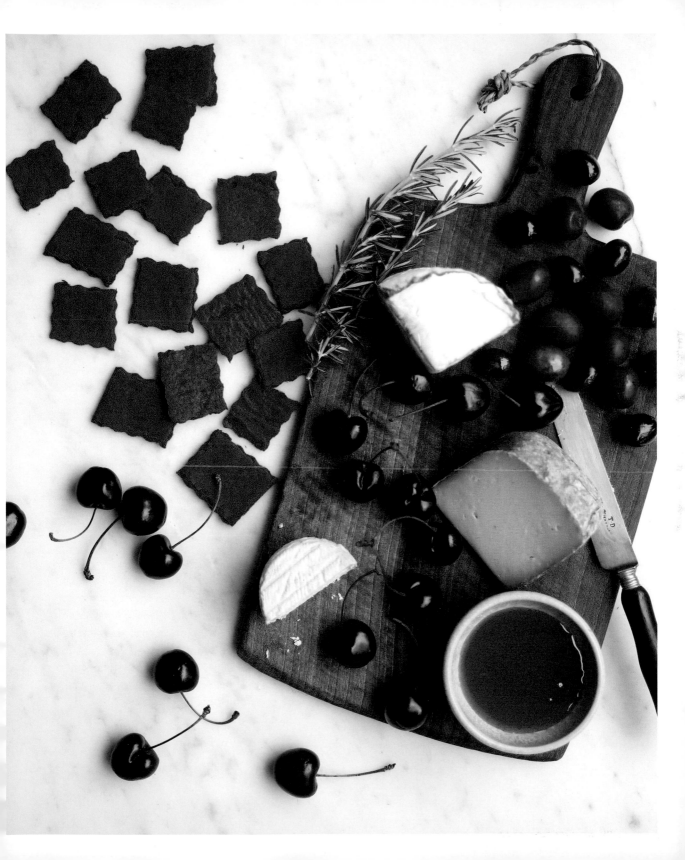

cinnamon oat crackers

MAKES ABOUT 30 CRACKERS | $0.51 PER SERVING

STARCH

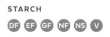

1 cup gluten-free oat flour (see page 189)

3 tablespoons ground chia seeds

⅛ teaspoon fine sea salt

6 tablespoons coconut sugar

1 teaspoon ground cinnamon

¼ cup coconut oil, melted

1 to 2 tablespoons water (just enough to make a dough)

These crackers are a healthier alternative to all the sweet "snack" crackers marketed to kids, like graham crackers and animal cookies. They are made with gluten-free oat flour for an allergy-friendly alternative that is safe for taking to school, and they are loaded with extra fiber and omega-3 fatty acids from the addition of chia seeds. They aren't supersweet like the store-bought variety, but you can always sprinkle a bit of extra coconut sugar and cinnamon on top before baking to satisfy any picky family members.

1   Preheat the oven to 350°F and line a baking sheet with parchment paper. In a large mixing bowl, combine the flour, chia seeds, salt, coconut sugar, cinnamon, coconut oil, and water and stir well to create a uniform dough.

2   Transfer the dough to the prepared baking sheet and top it with another sheet of parchment paper. Use a rolling pin to roll the dough into a thin layer, about ⅛ inch thick. The thinner you roll the dough, the crispier your crackers will get, and the faster they will cook. Gently remove the top layer of parchment paper and use a pizza cutter to cut the crackers into 1-inch squares.

3   Bake for 10 minutes, then remove the baking sheet from the oven and use a spatula to flip each cracker for even baking (they should easily split apart where you cut them).

4   Return the pan to the oven to bake until the crackers are dry and crisp, 5 to 10 minutes more (although it may take longer if your crackers are thicker). Be sure to watch the crackers closely toward the end of the baking time since the edge pieces will cook faster than the center pieces, and the crackers won't taste as good if they turn dark brown. Remove any pieces by the edge of the pan when they are done and continue cooking the center crackers until they are all dry. Allow the crackers to cool completely for the crispiest results. Store in an airtight container at room temperature for up to 1 week.

cashew queso

MAKES 2½ CUPS | $0.39 PER SERVING

This creamy queso tastes ridiculously similar to the popular dip made with a block of processed cheese and a can of diced tomatoes, but this dairy-free version gets its creaminess from raw cashews. Not only do cashews have a lower fat content than most other nuts, but they're also loaded with iron, magnesium, and antioxidants that can promote cardiovascular health. Paired with fresh lemon juice and tomatoes, which provide a healthy dose of vitamin C, this recipe is a party snack you can feel great about serving—and it will disappear before you know it! Serve with your favorite baked chips or crunchy sliced vegetables.

NUT/SEED/DRIED FRUIT

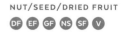

1 cup raw cashews, soaked in water for 2 hours and then drained

½ cup water

1 teaspoon fine sea salt

1½ tablespoons freshly squeezed lemon juice

3 tablespoons nutritional yeast

1 cup Fresh Pico de Gallo (page 188) or 1 (14-ounce) can diced tomatoes with green chiles

1 In a high-speed blender or food processor, combine the cashews, water, salt, lemon juice, and nutritional yeast and blend until completely smooth.

2 In a small saucepan, combine the mixture with the pico de gallo and gently warm over medium heat. It tastes the most authentic when warm! Store leftovers in an airtight container in the refrigerator for up to 5 days.

NOTE: Raw cashews have a very mild and neutral flavor that works well in this recipe. Try to avoid using roasted cashews, which have a stronger flavor.

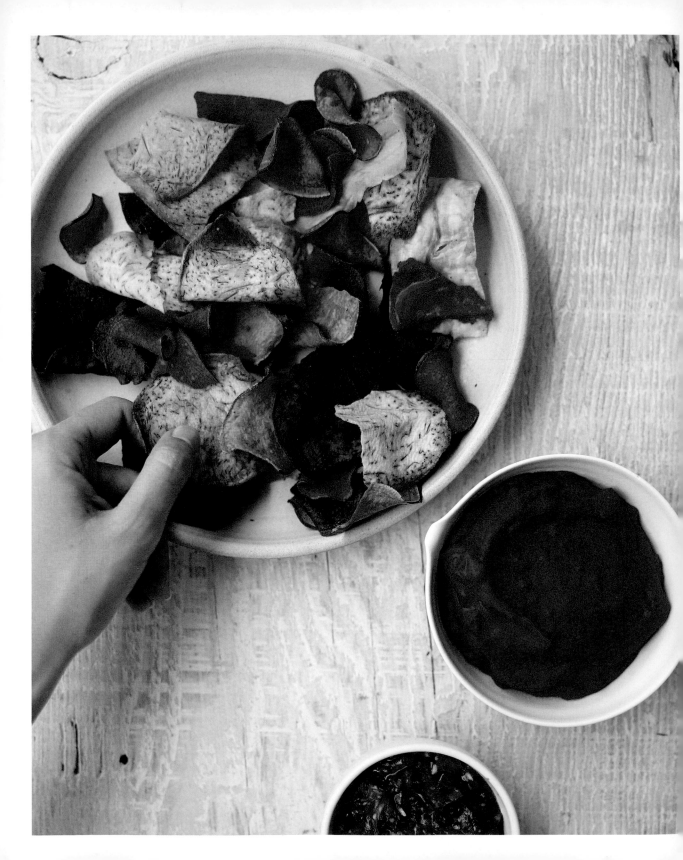

sweet potato queso

MAKES 2 CUPS | $0.40 PER SERVING

Similar to my Cashew Queso (page 97), this creamy sweet potato dip is perfect for nut-free households or for those who want a dip that is lower in fat. Sweet potatoes are brimming with nutrients, including beta-carotene, vitamin C, and potassium, and when paired with nutritional yeast, which is a complete source of vegetarian protein, this creamy, cheeselike sauce is a nutritional powerhouse. Serve it as a dip with your favorite baked chips or sliced vegetables at your next party or as a dairy-free topping for your favorite vegetables.

STARCH

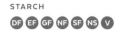

1 cup mashed sweet potato

½ cup water

1½ teaspoons fine sea salt

½ teaspoon chili powder

¼ cup nutritional yeast

1 teaspoon freshly squeezed lemon juice

1 cup Fresh Pico de Gallo (page 188)

1 In a high-speed blender, combine the sweet potato, water, salt, chili powder, nutritional yeast, and lemon juice and blend until completely smooth.

2 In a small saucepan, combine the mixture with the pico de gallo and gently warm over medium heat. Serve warm. Store leftovers in an airtight container in the refrigerator for up to 5 days.

NOTE: If you don't care for the flavor of sweet potatoes, you can easily substitute a Yukon gold potato with similarly delicious results.

mini pizza bites

MAKES 10 TO 12 PIECES | $0.27 PER SERVING

ANIMAL PROTEIN

10 to 12 small baby
bella mushrooms

⅓ cup pizza sauce
(no sugar added)

¼ cup grated Pecorino
Romano cheese

2 ounces goat cheddar,
shredded

Fresh basil, for garnish
(optional)

These bite-size appetizers remind me of my childhood-favorite freezer pizza bites. I recommend using homemade pizza sauce (page 186) for this recipe because it contains less moisture than traditional marinara sauce and will give you a more pizzalike result. Feel free to get creative with the toppings and pile on any favorites you like!

1   Preheat the oven to 350°F. Gently wipe each mushroom with a dry cloth to remove any dirt and remove the stem, keeping the rest of the mushroom intact. In a 10-inch oven-safe skillet, arrange the mushrooms in a single layer with the crevice facing up.

2   In a small bowl, stir together the pizza sauce and grated cheese, then spoon the filling into the center of each mushroom, using roughly 1 teaspoon per mushroom. Top with the shredded cheese (and any other pizza toppings you like) and bake until the mushrooms are tender, about 25 minutes.

3   Remove from the oven and top with fresh basil. Serve warm.

NOTE: These mushrooms would also be delicious filled with Zucchini Pesto (see page 133) in lieu of the pizza sauce.

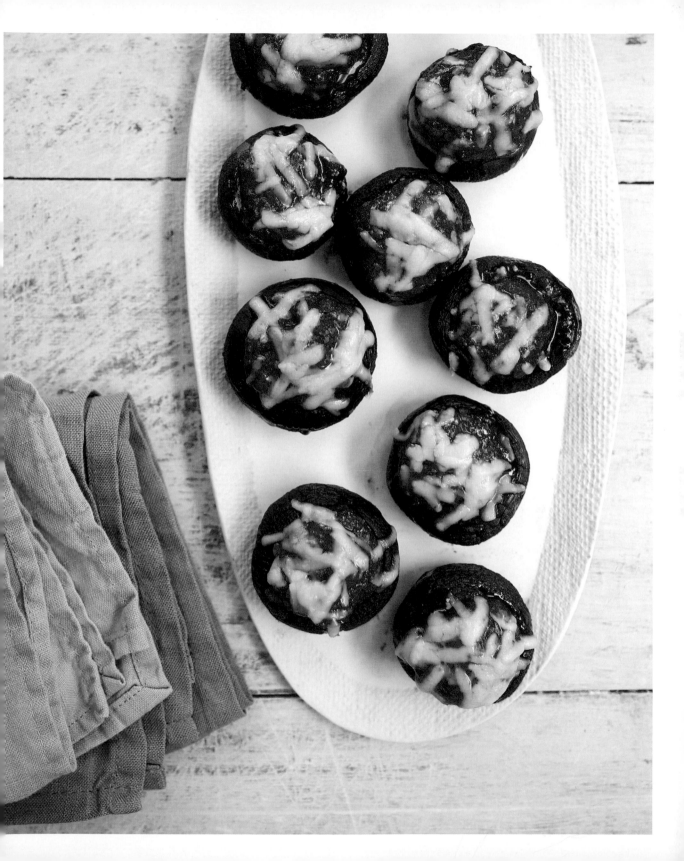

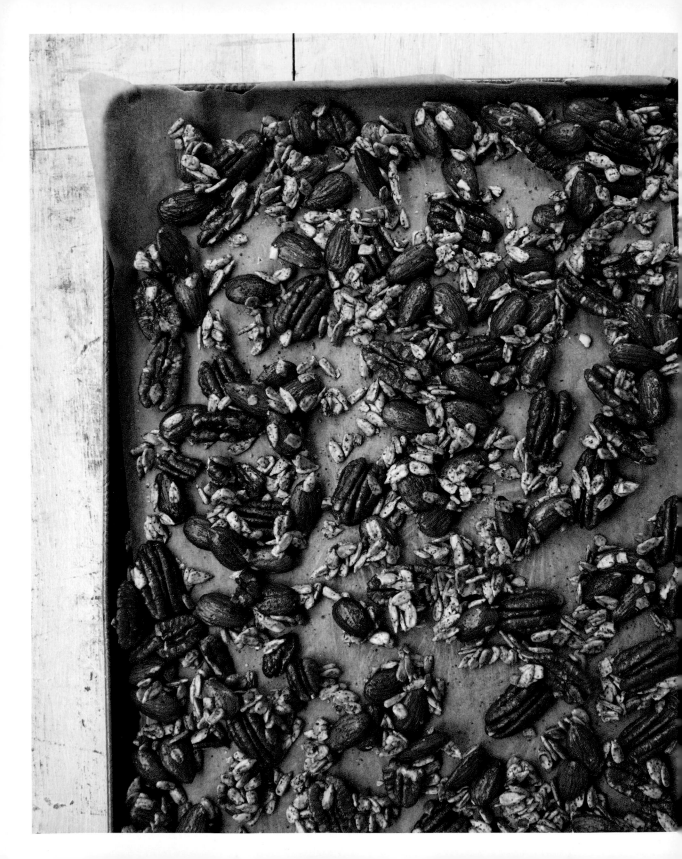

easy party mix

MAKES 2 CUPS | $0.44 PER SERVING

If you tend to crave that popular party mix, you are going to love this grain-free version. It tastes surprisingly similar to the kind made with rice cereal and is incredibly easy to prepare using any nuts or seeds you have on hand. Because this crispy mix can be stored at room temperature, it also makes a great snack on the go! Feel free to double the recipe because it will go fast.

1   Preheat the oven to 250°F and line a baking sheet with parchment paper.

2   In a large bowl, stir together the almonds, pecans, sunflower seeds, maple syrup, chili powder, garlic powder, and salt. Spread the mixture on the prepared baking sheet in a flat, single layer without too many clumps.

3   Bake for 35 minutes, then cool completely (the nuts will be crunchy once completely cool). Store in an airtight container at room temperature for up to 1 week or in the refrigerator for up to 2 weeks.

NUT/SEED/DRIED FRUIT

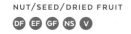

½ cup raw almonds

½ cup raw pecans

1 cup hulled sunflower seeds

1 tablespoon maple syrup

½ teaspoon chili powder

½ teaspoon garlic powder

¾ teaspoon fine sea salt

Cut Your Cancer Risk

The International Agency for Research on Cancer considers acrylamide to be a "probable human carcinogen," since it has been found to cause cancer in laboratory animals. This chemical is not added to food but is created naturally when certain foods are roasted, fried, or baked, particularly fries, potato chips, coffee, almonds, crackers, and bread. It is nearly impossible to avoid this chemical altogether, since it occurs naturally in a wide range of plant foods and animal products, but you can limit your exposure by using safer cooking methods, such as steaming and boiling, cooking susceptible foods at lower temperatures, and avoiding meats, vegetables, and starches that are darkly browned or charred. You'll notice that all of the recipes in this book that call for heating raw nuts are kept to temperatures of 250°F or lower to avoid browning and to reduce the potential formation of acrylamide.

southwest lettuce wraps
with sweet cilantro dressing

SERVES 4 | $1.71 PER SERVING

STARCH

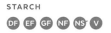

SWEET CILANTRO DRESSING

2 tablespoons extra-virgin olive oil

¼ cup water

¼ ripe Hass avocado

2 tablespoons raw apple cider vinegar

1 tablespoon freshly squeezed lime juice

2 tablespoons raw honey

½ cup tightly packed fresh cilantro

1 tablespoon seeded minced jalapeño chile

1 teaspoon minced fresh ginger

1 teaspoon coconut oil

½ red onion, chopped

1 red bell pepper, chopped

1 ripe Hass avocado

1½ cups cooked black beans (see page 78) or 1 (15-ounce) can, rinsed and drained

2 green onions, white and green parts, chopped

½ teaspoon sea salt

1 tablespoon freshly squeezed lime juice

1 head of butter lettuce, for serving

These tasty wraps were inspired by a college favorite of mine—the deep-fried avocado egg rolls from the Cheesecake Factory. What sets these wraps apart is an amazing sweet cilantro dipping sauce, paired with a creamy avocado filling. Instead of making oily egg rolls, serve this delicious filling in buttery lettuce cups and drench it in the sweet cilantro dressing for a fast and fresh experience you can enjoy at home.

1   To prepare the dressing: In a high-speed blender, combine the olive oil, water, avocado, vinegar, lime juice, honey, cilantro, jalapeño, and ginger and blend until completely smooth. Set aside in the refrigerator to let the flavors meld.

2   In a skillet, melt the coconut oil over medium-high heat and sauté the onion and bell pepper until tender, 8 to 10 minutes.

3   Meanwhile, in a large mixing bowl, mash the avocado and add the beans, green onions, salt, and lime juice. Once the veggies are done cooking, add them to the bowl, too, and stir well to combine. You can leave the beans whole, or use the back of a fork to mash them a bit, depending on how you prefer the texture. Taste the filling and adjust any seasoning, if necessary.

4   Spoon the filling into lettuce leaves and generously spoon the dressing over the top just before serving. Store leftover filling in an airtight container in the refrigerator for up to 2 days, but keep in mind that the avocado will start to brown and make the filling look visually less appealing. Store leftover dressing in the refrigerator for up to 4 days; it makes a fantastic salad topper.

NOTE: If you don't mind the flavor of raw onion, you can skip the sautéing step and add the onion and bell pepper right into the filling for a faster alternative.

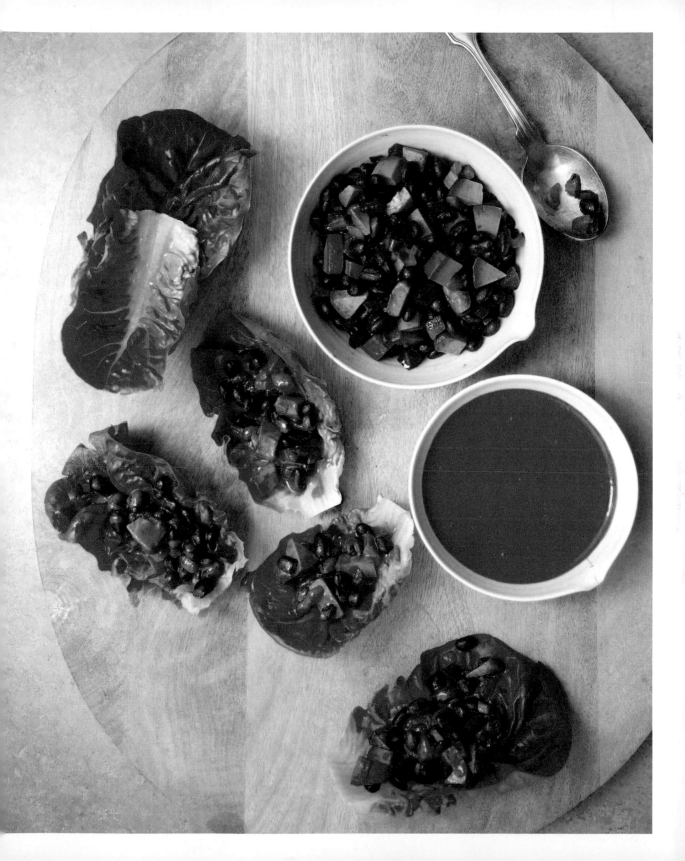

white bean & rosemary dip

MAKES ABOUT 2 CUPS | $0.28 PER SERVING

STARCH

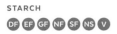

1½ cups cooked cannellini beans (see page 78) or 1 (15-ounce) can, rinsed and drained

½ small zucchini, peeled and diced

1 tablespoon freshly squeezed lemon juice

2 cloves garlic, minced

½ teaspoon fine sea salt

2 tablespoons extra-virgin olive oil

1 teaspoon minced fresh rosemary

Freshly ground black pepper

This dip was inspired by a pizza restaurant in Kansas City called Spin! Pizza, which serves the best white bean hummus I've ever tasted. My picky toddler son will eat it straight with a spoon! This version is properly combined for easier digestion and still has a great flavor that is perfect for dipping with veggies or your favorite crackers or flatbread. You can leave the peel on the zucchini if you prefer, but keep in mind that it will give this dip a slightly greenish hue.

1   In a food processor, combine the beans, zucchini, lemon juice, garlic, salt, olive oil, and rosemary; season with pepper; and blend until relatively smooth—it's okay if there is still a bit of texture. (If the dip is too thick, add 1 to 2 tablespoons water and blend until your desired consistency is reached.) Adjust the seasonings, if necessary. Serve immediately. Store leftovers in an airtight container in the refrigerator for up to 1 week.

zucchini hummus

MAKES 1½ CUPS | $0.67 PER SERVING

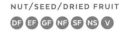

15-MINUTE PREP

This hummus is a weekly staple in our home. Traditional hummus is not properly combined, so instead of using chickpeas for the base, this recipe uses zucchini, which is loaded with vitamin C, magnesium, potassium, folate, and fiber to help keep your digestion running smoothly. Combined with calcium-rich tahini, this recipe is a delicious snack to help you meet your daily nutrient needs, particularly when served with sliced vegetables. Serve chilled with your favorite sliced vegetables.

NUT/SEED/DRIED FRUIT

DF EF GF NF SF NS V

1 cup diced zucchini

⅓ cup raw tahini (see Note, page 56)

1 to 2 tablespoons freshly squeezed lemon juice

1 clove garlic, minced

½ teaspoon sea salt

2 teaspoons ground cumin

1   In a small food processor or high-speed blender, combine the zucchini, tahini, 1 tablespoon of lemon juice, garlic, salt, and cumin and blend until smooth and creamy. Adjust any seasoning, adding another tablesppon of lemon juice if desired, then chill in the refrigerator for 1 hour before serving. Store leftovers in an airtight container in the refrigerator for up to 5 days.

loaded nacho dip

SERVES 8 | $0.77 PER SERVING

STARCH

(DF) (EF) (GF) (NF) (SF) (NS) (V)

BEAN LAYER

3 cups cooked black beans (see page 78) or 2 (15-ounce) cans, rinsed and drained

½ teaspoon fine sea salt

½ teaspoon ground cumin

½ teaspoon chili powder

½ teaspoon garlic powder

½ teaspoon onion powder

¼ cup water

"CHEESE" SAUCE

1 cup steamed and mashed Yukon gold potatoes

½ cup water

¼ cup nutritional yeast

1 tablespoon freshly squeezed lemon juice

1 teaspoon onion powder

1 teaspoon fine sea salt

Guacamole (page 188), for topping

Fresh Pico de Gallo (page 188) or salsa, for topping

Chopped green onions, for garnish

This dip is inspired by the popular 7-layer dip you may have encountered at parties, but this version is entirely plant-based for a healthier alternative. While it doesn't take too long to prepare each layer from scratch, you are welcome to speed up the process by using prepared guacamole and pico de gallo from your local supermarket. Paired with a spicy black bean layer and creamy "cheese" sauce, this dip will make you feel as if you're eating nachos when you serve it with Baked Parsnip Chips (page 114) or your favorite chips.

1   To prepare the bean layer: In a food processor, combine the beans, salt, cumin, chili powder, garlic powder, onion powder, and water and process until a uniform texture is achieved. Spread the beans evenly over the bottom of a 9-inch square dish.

2   To prepare the "cheese" sauce: In a high-speed blender, combine the potatoes, water, yeast, lemon juice, onion powder, and salt and blend until completely smooth and creamy. Pour over the bean layer.

3   Spoon the guacamole over the "cheese" sauce layer. Top the guacamole with the pico de gallo and garnish with chopped green onions. Serve immediately, or chill in the refrigerator for up to 48 hours, but keep the dip tightly wrapped, because the guacamole will start to brown due to oxidation.

NOTE: If serving this dip with corn chips, be sure to shop for organic varieties to ensure the corn has not been genetically modified or sprayed with insecticides that threaten the bee population.

MAKE IT AHEAD: If you would like to prepare this dish in advance, store the guacamole and pico de gallo separately, and add those two layers on top just before serving. This will prevent the guacamole from browning and the dip from becoming soggy.

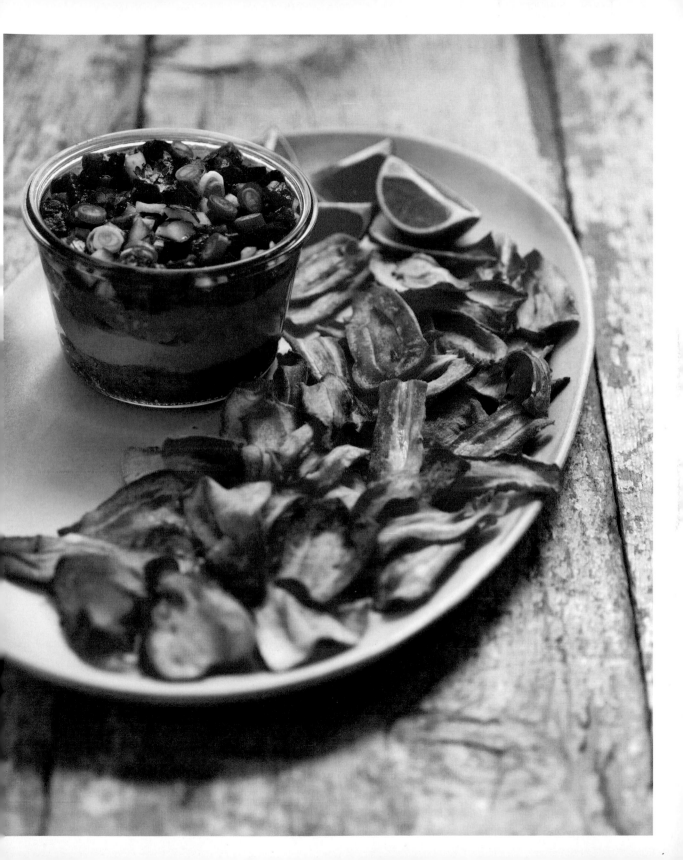

garden spring rolls
with creamy tahini dipping sauce

MAKES 8 ROLLS | $1.95 PER SERVING

NUT/SEED/DRIED FRUIT

DF EF GF NF

**CREAMY TAHINI
DIPPING SAUCE**

¼ cup raw tahini

2 tablespoons extra-
virgin olive oil

1 tablespoon freshly
squeezed lemon juice

1 tablespoon tamari
(gluten-free soy sauce)

3 tablespoons raw
honey

1 clove garlic, minced

1-inch knob of fresh
ginger, peeled and
chopped

¼ teaspoon salt

¼ teaspoon red pepper
flakes

¼ cup water

SPRING ROLLS

8 sheets of rice paper
(see Note)

16 leaves romaine
lettuce

2 green bell peppers,
sliced

1 cucumber, sliced

2 ripe Hass avocados,
sliced

4 carrots, shredded

These rolls were inspired by an offering in the prepared sushi section at my local grocery store, where they sell prepared garden vegetable wraps, which are essentially an assortment of raw salad vegetables wrapped in rice paper and served with an addictive peanut dipping sauce. The store-bought rolls could easily become an expensive habit, so this recipe is a more affordable and peanut-free alternative. The rice paper isn't perfectly combined with the tahini-based dipping sauce, but if you find this combination bothers you, you can simply omit the rice paper and serve these rolls as lettuce wraps instead.

1   To prepare the sauce: In a high-speed blender, combine the tahini, olive oil, lemon juice, tamari, honey, garlic, ginger, salt, red pepper flakes, and water and blend until smooth. (Add additional water if you would like a thinner consistency.) Store in the refrigerator for up to 4 days.

2   To prepare the spring rolls: Wet a sheet of rice paper with warm water and lay it on a flat work surface, such as a cutting board. Arrange 2 lettuce leaves, several bell pepper and cucumber slices, one-fourth of an avocado, and some carrots in the center of the rice paper, making sure not to get too close to the edges of the paper.

3   Fold the sides of the rice paper in toward the middle, then grab the bottom of the rice paper and roll it toward the top, as if you were rolling up a burrito. The paper should be flexible and sticky, so when you get to the end it should automatically stick together and seal shut.

4   Use a sharp knife to slice the roll sushi-style, if you like, then serve with the chilled dipping sauce. These rolls are best served fresh, but will keep in an airtight container in the refrigerator for up to 48 hours.

NOTE: Both brown rice and white rice paper work equally well in this recipe. While brown rice has a reputation for being "healthier," the white rice paper usually has fewer ingredients and is slightly easier to work with.

date energy bites

MAKES ABOUT 24 PIECES | $0.20 PER SERVING

15-MINUTE PREP
KID-FRIENDLY
FREEZER-FRIENDLY

I always have a batch of these bite-size treats on hand, since they're quick to prepare, taste like dessert, and are loaded with nutrients. You can use any nut or seed combination you happen to have on hand, but I particularly love using walnuts because they contain the omega-3 fatty acid alpha-linolenic acid, which is an anti-inflammatory agent and has been shown to reduce the risk of heart attacks.[1] Paired with low-glycemic dates, which are a good source of calcium and iron, these treats are a guilt-free snack you can enjoy at any time of the day!

NUT/SEED/DRIED FRUIT

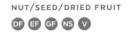

2 cups walnuts or other nut/seed of choice

1 cup shredded unsweetened coconut

About 16 soft Medjool dates, pitted

1 teaspoon vanilla extract

½ teaspoon sea salt

1   Line a baking sheet or plate with parchment paper.

2   In a large food processor fitted with an "S" blade, process the walnuts and coconut until crumbly. Add the dates, vanilla, and salt and process again until a sticky, uniform batter is formed. (If the mixture isn't sticking together, add 1 tablespoon water and process again until sticky.)

3   Scoop the dough by heaping tablespoons, then roll between your hands to form balls. Arrange the balls in a single layer on the prepared baking sheet, then place in the freezer to set for 1 hour before serving. Store in an airtight container in the refrigerator for up to 2 weeks or in the freezer for up to 6 months. (They taste great directly from the freezer, too!) These balls will soften if left at room temperature for too long, but if you don't mind the softer texture, they make an easy and delicious snack on the go.

NOTE: For a gourmetlike truffle, roll these balls in raw cacao powder or shredded coconut before chilling.

nut-free chewy granola bars

MAKES 12 BARS | $0.38 PER SERVING

SPECIAL TREAT

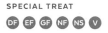

2 cups rolled oats

½ teaspoon ground cinnamon

½ teaspoon sea salt

½ cup raisins

½ cup maple syrup

½ cup unsweetened and unsalted sunflower seed butter

While these granola bars aren't perfectly combined, they are an upgrade from the huge selection of processed and refined sugar–filled snacks on the market. Sunflower seed butter helps keep these bars chewy and nut-free for an easy school-safe snack, but feel free to use your favorite nut butter of choice if staying nut-free isn't essential for your situation. If you can't easily locate sunflower butter in your local store, you can easily make it at home using the recipe on page 187.

1   Line a 9-inch square baking dish with parchment paper. Set aside.

2   In a large mixing bowl, combine the oats, cinnamon, salt, and raisins and stir to combine.

3   In a small saucepan, bring the maple syrup to a boil over medium-high heat and set a timer to let it boil for 1 minute. Remove the boiled syrup from the heat and immediately stir in the sunflower seed butter.

4   Pour the heated mixture over the oats and stir well to evenly coat. It will be sticky, so be sure to use a sturdy spoon to do the job. Transfer the mixture to the prepared baking dish and spread it evenly with a spatula. The mixture needs to be pressed together very firmly, so top it with another sheet of parchment paper and use your hands and all of your body weight to firmly press into the bottom of the pan. Remove the top layer of parchment paper and place in the freezer to set, about 1 hour.

5   After the mixture is firm, remove from the freezer and slice into 12 bars using a sharp knife. For the best shelf life, store the bars individually wrapped in the refrigerator for up to 1 month or in the freezer for up to 6 months, but for the best texture, allow them to come to room temperature before eating. The frozen bars will thaw in about an hour, so they make a great snack on the go!

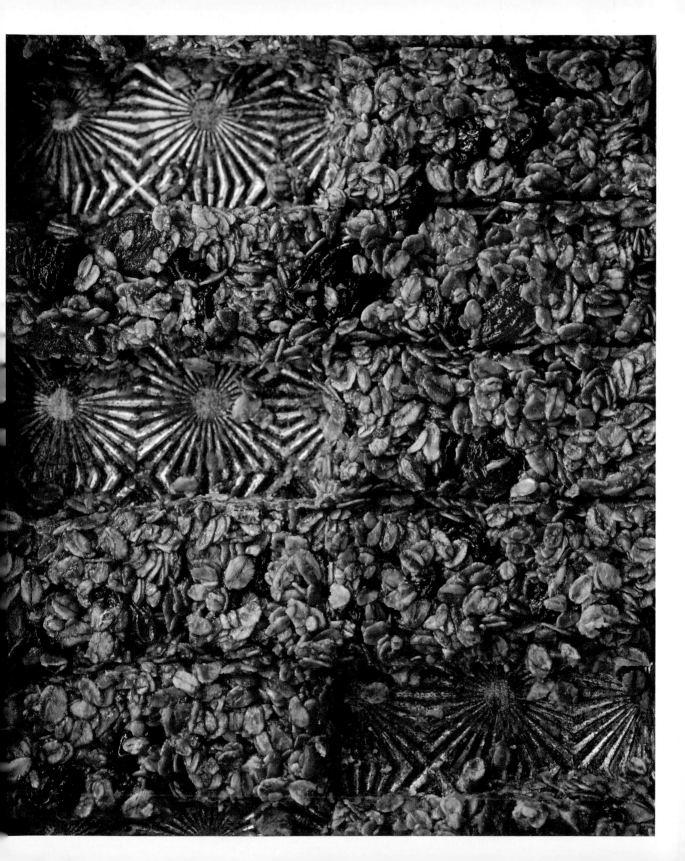

baked parsnip chips

SERVES 2 | $0.64 PER SERVING

NEUTRAL

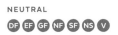

1 large parsnip

2 teaspoons
coconut oil, melted

Sea salt

These chips (pictured on page 109) crisp up just like potato chips, but parsnips are loaded with more potassium and vitamin C than potatoes for a more nutrient-dense snack. Baking these chips at a lower temperature helps them bake evenly, letting you avoid any soft or chewy centers, so be patient—they are worth it!

1   Preheat the oven to 250°F and line a large baking sheet with parchment paper.

2   Slice the parsnip diagonally using a mandoline to create larger slices. (No need to peel the parsnip first.) You want the slices to be paper thin, about 1⁄16 inch thick. The thinner you slice them, the crispier they will get, and using a mandoline will help keep the slices uniform so they will bake in roughly the same amount of time.

3   In a large mixing bowl, toss the parsnips with the coconut oil and arrange them on the prepared baking sheet. (Depending on the size of your parsnip, you may need a second baking sheet to cook all of the slices at once.) Sprinkle with salt.

4   Bake for 45 to 60 minutes, until golden and crisp. Check on the chips at 30 minutes and remove any small pieces that are brown, since the smaller and thinner pieces will cook more quickly.

5   Return the baking sheet to the oven and bake the remaining chips; be sure to check on them every 5 to 10 minutes to remove any golden chips so they don't burn. Allow the chips to cool completely before serving for the crispiest results. Store leftovers in an airtight container at room temperature for up to 3 days.

crispy garlic chickpeas

SERVES 4 | $0.26 PER SERVING

This crunchy snack is allergy-friendly and packs a satisfying 5 grams of protein and 4 grams of fiber into each large handful. While the chickpeas do take a while to bake, they require only about 10 minutes of hands-on time to prepare, making them an easy snack to concoct while you multitask around the house. Enjoy them as a quick snack on the go or as crunchy "croutons" over the Avocado Caesar Salad on page 73.

STARCH

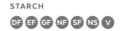

1½ cups cooked chickpeas (see page 78) or 1 (15-ounce) can, rinsed and drained

1 tablespoon extra-virgin olive oil

½ teaspoon fine sea salt

½ teaspoon garlic powder

½ teaspoon onion powder

1   Preheat the oven to 350°F. If using canned chickpeas, place them in a towel and gently rub dry. (It's okay if a few skins fall off.)

2   Arrange the chickpeas in a single layer on a rimmed baking sheet, drizzle with the olive oil, and shake the pan vigorously to coat the beans. Sprinkle the salt, garlic powder, and onion powder over the top and shake again.

3   Bake for 30 minutes, then shake the chickpeas to flip them for even crisping. Return to the oven to continue baking until they are fragrant and golden in color, 10 to 15 minutes more. Allow to cool completely before serving. Store in an airtight container at room temperature for up to 48 hours or in the refrigerator for up to 1 week. If the chickpeas become soft when stored, reheat them in the oven for another 15 minutes to crisp them.

Cooking with Olive Oil

I often use coconut oil in any heated recipe because it is high in saturated fat, which makes it a very stable cooking oil. However, studies have shown that extra-virgin olive oil can also withstand quite a bit of heat (up to 36 hours at 350°F) while still retaining most of its nutritional properties,[2] so if you don't care for the taste of coconut oil, feel free to use extra-virgin olive oil in its place. Note that this is not the case for no-bake recipes, in which the saturated fat is essential to the texture of the final product. Don't be tempted to use olive oil in a dessert or snack bar, unless it is specifically called for.

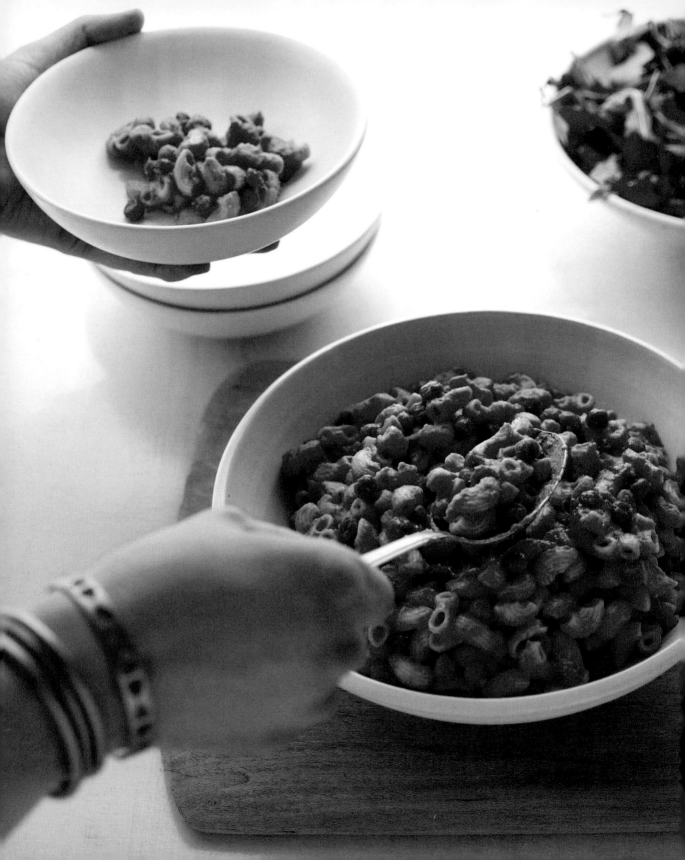

6 COMFORT FOOD & CASSEROLES

sloppy joe–stuffed sweet potatoes

SERVES 4 TO 6 | $1.39 TO $2.09 PER SERVING

STARCH

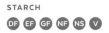

1 tablespoon
coconut oil

1 yellow onion, chopped

1 green bell pepper,
chopped

2 cloves garlic, minced

1½ cups tomato puree
(strained tomatoes)

Fine sea salt

1½ tablespoons Dijon
mustard

1 to 2 tablespoons
maple syrup

1½ cups water

1 teaspoon chili powder

1 cup dried red lentils

4 to 6 cooked sweet
potatoes (see page 14)
or your favorite
sandwich buns

Parsley and green
onions, for garnish
(optional)

Sloppy Joes are a classic childhood favorite, and this fresh vegetarian version is loaded with fiber, lean protein, and minerals such as potassium, calcium, and zinc. Unlike other varieties of lentils that take much longer to cook, red lentils are tender in just 20 minutes, and they are the perfect vehicle for this sweet and spicy sauce. Served over a baked sweet potato, this dish is comforting, filling, and ultra-nourishing, but you can also serve it on your favorite bun to please any picky eaters.

1   In a large pot, melt the coconut oil over medium heat and sauté the onion, bell pepper, and garlic until tender, 8 to 10 minutes. Add the tomato puree, 1½ teaspoons salt, mustard, 1 tablespoon of the maple syrup, the water, chili powder, and lentils and bring the mixture to a rolling boil.

2   Lower the heat to a simmer and cover to cook until the lentils are very tender, about 20 minutes. Stir intermittently through the simmering process to make sure none of the lentils sticks to the bottom of the pot. When the lentils are tender, adjust any seasonings as needed, adding up to 1 tablespoon maple syrup to taste.

3   Slice the sweet potatoes in half lengthwise and gently mash with a fork, sprinkle with salt, and spoon the filling over the top and garnish, or simply serve the filling in your favorite sandwich bun.

MAKE IT AHEAD: Use the Freezer or Slow/Pressure Cooker Method on page 15.

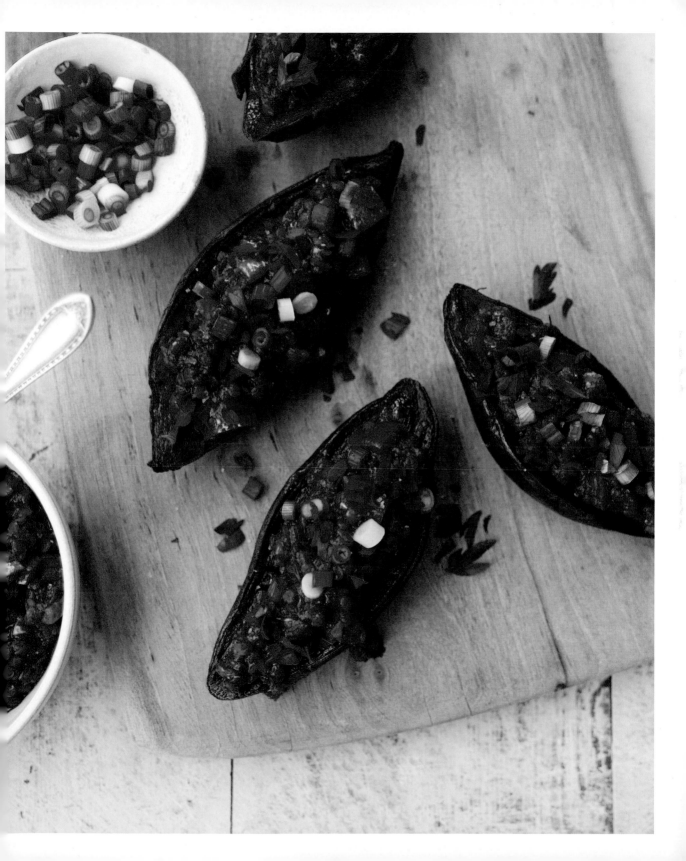

spinach & artichoke "pasta" bake

SERVES 4 TO 6 | $2.11 TO $3.24 PER SERVING

ANIMAL PROTEIN

1 tablespoon butter or coconut oil

½ yellow onion, chopped

1 clove garlic, minced

1 spaghetti squash, cooked (see page 14)

12 ounces frozen artichoke hearts, thawed and coarsely chopped

2 cups fresh baby spinach, chopped

2 teaspoons fine sea salt

1 cup plain goat's milk yogurt

¾ cup grated Pecorino Romano cheese

Freshly ground black pepper

This recipe involves a little bit of planning ahead, but it comes together easily when you're prepared. Be sure to thaw the frozen artichoke hearts in the refrigerator the night before you plan on making this dish, or you can speed up the process, as I do when I forget to thaw them, by placing them in a bowl of hot water. With a creamy texture and cheesy flavor reminiscent of the popular party dip, this vegetable-based "pasta" dish is sure to be a hit.

1   Preheat the oven to 350°F. In a skillet, melt the butter over medium heat and sauté the onion and garlic until tender, 8 to 10 minutes.

2   Transfer the onion and garlic to a large mixing bowl, then use the tines of a fork to scrape the cooked spaghetti squash "noodles" into the bowl. Add the artichoke hearts, spinach, salt, yogurt, and ½ cup of the grated cheese. Season with pepper and stir well to combine.

3   Transfer the mixture to a 9 by 13-inch glass baking dish and use a spatula to smooth the top. Sprinkle the remaining ¼ cup cheese over the top.

4   Bake until heated through, about 30 minutes. Serve warm. Store leftovers in an airtight container in the refrigerator for up to 5 days.

NOTE: I love using frozen artichokes because they have the same meaty texture and mild flavor as the fresh variety but require almost zero work to prepare—perfect for busy people who care about eating well. Canned artichokes have a very salty and preserved flavor that can be overpowering, but if that is your only option, be sure to rinse them well and decrease the salt in this recipe by ½ teaspoon to compensate.

MISS THE MEAT? Add your favorite high-quality meat to this properly combined dish. Simply cook the raw meat with the onions in step 1 and drain any excess juices before moving on to step 2.

MAKE IT AHEAD: Assemble the casserole and freeze it for up to 6 months before baking. To heat, thaw in the fridge overnight, then place the dish in a cold oven. Turn on the oven to 350°F and bake until heated through, about 1 hour and 15 minutes.

philly cheesesteak–stuffed spaghetti squash

SERVES 2 | $3.76 PER SERVING

This dish is the ultimate combination of two comfort foods—Philly cheesesteak sandwiches and pasta. All of the flavor in this popular sandwich is in the filling, so I've tossed it with vegetable-based noodles for a lighter, yet tasty alternative. When spaghetti squash isn't in season, you can also use zucchini "noodles" or any other veggies you like. A topping of cheese makes this dish ultra-comforting, but those following a Paleo or vegan diet can easily omit it. If you feel the need for animal protein, you're welcome to add meat to this properly combined dish.

ANIMAL PROTEIN

2 teaspoons butter or coconut oil

1 yellow onion, thinly sliced

1 red bell pepper, coarsely chopped

1 green bell pepper, coarsely chopped

8 ounces mushrooms, sliced

1 (3-pound) spaghetti squash, cooked (see page 14)

1 teaspoon garlic powder

1½ teaspoons fine sea salt

Pinch of cayenne pepper

2 to 3 ounces goat cheddar, shredded (optional)

Freshly ground black pepper

1 Preheat the broiler. In a large, deep skillet or Dutch oven, melt the butter over medium heat and sauté the onion and both bell peppers until the onion turns translucent, about 8 minutes. Add the mushrooms and sauté until they are tender, about 5 minutes more.

2 Use the tines of a fork to scrape the spaghetti squash strands out of the cooked squash. (Use an oven mitt to hold the squash to avoid burning your hands.) Reserve the scraped shells.

3 Transfer the cooked "noodles" to the pan with the sautéed bell peppers and mushrooms, and add the garlic powder, salt, and cayenne. Stir well to make sure the seasoning is distributed evenly. Taste the "pasta" and adjust any seasonings, as needed. Scoop the cooked veggies into the reserved shells and top them generously with the cheese. Place the shells on a baking sheet under the broiler until the cheese is bubbly, 2 to 3 minutes, then season with pepper. Serve warm. Store leftovers in an airtight container in the refrigerator for up to 3 days.

MISS THE MEAT? Add your favorite high-quality steak or chicken to this properly combined dish. Just sauté it in step 2 with the onion and bell peppers and drain any excess juices.

MAKE IT AHEAD: You can cook one or more spaghetti squash ahead of time and store them in an airtight container in the refrigerator for up to 1 week. You can add the cold noodles just as you would the hot noodles in this recipe—it will just take a few more minutes of sautéing to warm them up. Using this method, this meal can be ready in just about 20 minutes!

butternut mac 'n' cheese

SERVES 4 TO 6 | $0.82 TO $1.23 PER SERVING

STARCH

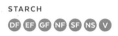

1 pound gluten-free
macaroni or shell pasta

1 cup fresh or thawed
from frozen shelled
peas

BUTTERNUT SQUASH
SAUCE

1 tablespoon
coconut oil

½ yellow onion,
chopped

1 clove garlic, minced

1 pound fresh or frozen
butternut squash
chunks

1¾ cups water

¼ cup nutritional yeast

2 teaspoons fine
sea salt

½ teaspoon
chili powder

1 tablespoon freshly
squeezed lemon juice

2 cups fresh baby
spinach, chopped
(optional)

2 to 4 cups leftover
roasted or sautéed
vegetables (optional)

While the cashew-based "cheese" sauce in my first book is wildly popular, it's not allergy-friendly or properly combined when served over high-quality pasta. So, this vegetable-based sauce is a delicious alternative for those who want a low-fat dish with a sneaky serving of veggies. It tastes better than any boxed version I've tried and has an authentic orange color without using any chemical additives or dyes. While this recipe won't necessarily fool everyone into thinking they are eating cheese, it won't stop them from going back for second helpings!

1   In a large pot, cook the pasta according to the package directions, adding the peas during the last 5 minutes of the cooking time.

2   To prepare the sauce: While the pasta is cooking, in a separate large pot, melt the coconut oil over medium-high heat and sauté the onion and garlic until they start to soften, about 5 minutes. Add the squash and 1 cup of the water and bring to a boil. Stir the veggies, lower the heat to a simmer, and cover the pot to cook the vegetables until tender, about 20 minutes.

3   Remove the lid and make sure the butternut squash is fork-tender. Simmer off any remaining liquid, then transfer the cooked vegetables to a high-speed blender. Add the remaining ¾ cup water, nutritional yeast, salt, chili powder, and lemon juice and blend until completely smooth. (Be sure to leave the vent in your blender lid open to prevent the steam pressure from building up—it could blow the lid off your blender and cause burns. Instead, loosely cover the vent with a thin dish towel to prevent splattering.)

4   Drain the tender pasta and peas and toss them with the butternut sauce in a large pot over medium heat to warm up everything. At this point, you can stir in the spinach, which will wilt quickly when stirred, or roasted vegetables. Taste and adjust any seasoning. Serve warm. Store leftovers in an airtight container in the refrigerator for up to 4 days.

MAKE IT AHEAD: Prepare and freeze this sauce up to 6 months in advance. Pour the sauce into ice-cube trays for easy portioning and reheating; you can stir the cubes directly into freshly cooked pasta when you need a quick meal.

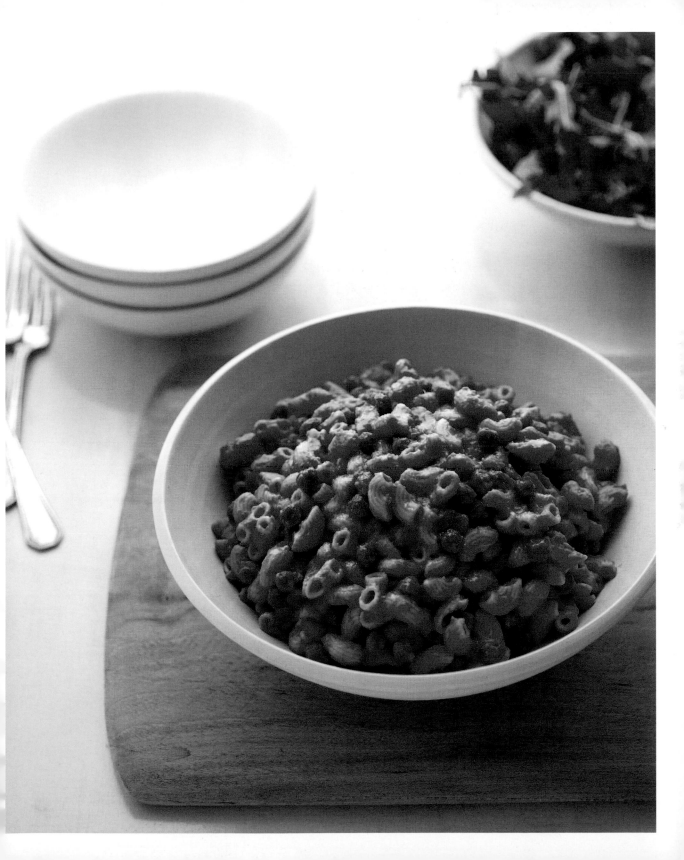

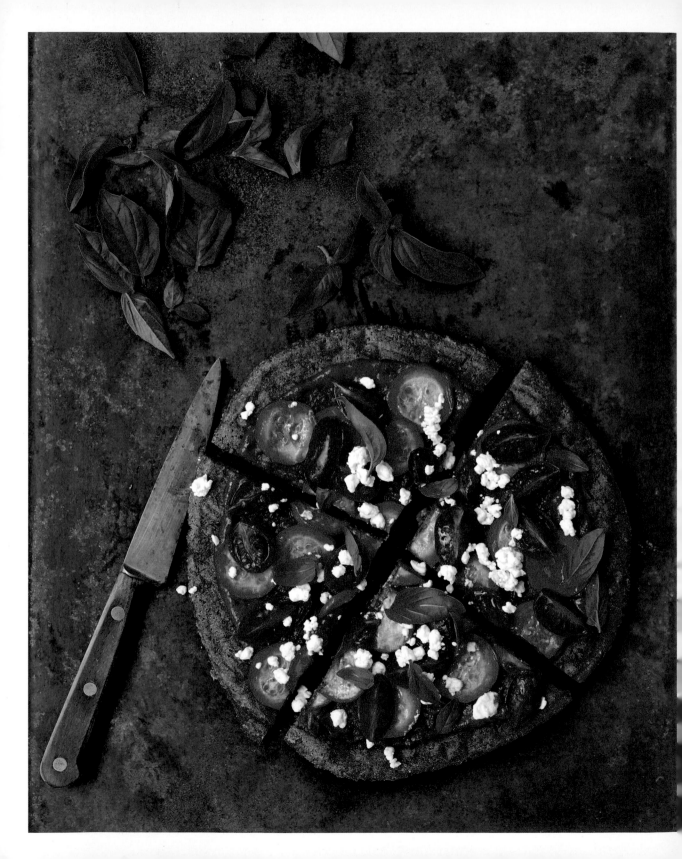

overnight quinoa pizza

MAKES ONE 10-INCH PIZZA | $0.93 PER SERVING

This gluten-free pizza crust is a protein-rich alternative to wheat-based crusts, boasts a sneaky serving of veggies in each bite, and can be customized by adding any of your favorite seasonings. The preparation doesn't take long, but it does help if you soak the quinoa ahead of time to soften it and remove any bitterness. Quinoa can withstand quite a bit of soaking, so feel free to place the quinoa in a bowl of water in the refrigerator the night before you plan to make this or in the morning before you go to work. This crust was deemed by several of my taste testers to be the "best and easiest gluten-free pizza crust" they've ever had. I hope you feel the same way!

STARCH

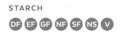

¾ cup quinoa, soaked for at least 8 hours or up to overnight in the refrigerator

½ cup peeled and chopped zucchini

½ teaspoon fine sea salt

½ teaspoon garlic powder

½ teaspoon baking soda

1 teaspoon apple cider vinegar

Your favorite veggie toppings, such as Zucchini Pesto (see page 133), roasted tomatoes, red onions, and bell peppers

1   Preheat the oven to 400°F and line a large baking sheet with parchment paper. For extra stick-prevention, grease the top of the parchment paper.

2   Drain and rinse the quinoa, then combine it with the zucchini, salt, garlic powder, baking soda, and vinegar in a blender and blend until a thick and smooth batter is formed. (If you need to add a splash of water to help it blend, that's okay.)

3   Use a spatula to spread and smooth the batter into a large circle, 10 to 12 inches in diameter, on the prepared baking sheet.

4   Bake for 15 minutes, then use the parchment paper to flip the crust and bake until the crust is dry, 5 to 10 minutes more depending on thickness. Top the crust as desired, then return to the oven and bake until the toppings are heated through, another 8 to 10 minutes. Slice and serve warm. Store leftover pizza in an airtight container in the refrigerator for up to 4 days.

MAKE IT AHEAD: This baked pizza crust freezes well, so you can prepare several crusts at once and freeze them for up to 3 months for a quick pizza night in the future. To reheat, simply remove the crust from the freezer and top it directly with your favorite toppings. (No need to thaw the crust first.) Bake at 400°F until the toppings are piping hot, 18 to 20 minutes.

cauliflower baked ziti

SERVES 4 | $3.07 PER SERVING

ANIMAL PROTEIN

1 head of cauliflower, cut into florets and chopped

2½ cups Pizza Sauce (page 186)

4 eggs

⅓ cup grated Pecorino Romano cheese

½ teaspoon fine sea salt

2 cups fresh baby spinach

2 ounces goat cheddar, shredded

If you're not familiar with baked ziti, it features all of the flavors of lasagna without the extra layering work. This dish is based on that idea, but instead of cooking pasta as you would for the traditional version, you'll use cauliflower as a lower-carb and higher-nutrient alternative. All of my taste testers, even self-proclaimed cauliflower haters, were surprised that this dish tasted like lasagna and not at all like cauliflower!

1 In a large Dutch oven, combine the cauliflower and pizza sauce and stir well to coat. Bring the sauce to a boil over medium-high heat and, once bubbling, lower the heat to a simmer and cover the pot to let the cauliflower cook until fork-tender, about 15 minutes.

2 Preheat the oven to 350°F. In a medium bowl, beat together the eggs, grated cheese, and salt. Set aside.

3 After the cauliflower is tender, stir in the spinach and simmer to cook off any excess moisture in the pot, to ensure that the final result isn't watery. Remove the pot from the heat and stir in the egg and cheese mixture. Top with the shredded cheese.

4 Bake for 30 minutes, until the eggs have set and the cheese is bubbly on top. Allow the dish to cool for 10 minutes, then serve warm. Store leftovers in an airtight container in the refrigerator for up to 5 days.

MISS THE MEAT? You are welcome to add your favorite high-quality meat to this properly combined dish. Simply sauté the meat in a separate pan while the cauliflower is cooking, then drain well and mix it in during step #3.

MAKE IT AHEAD: You can prepare this dish as a freezer meal by beating together the pizza sauce, eggs, cheese, and salt in a large bowl, then stirring in the raw cauliflower and spinach. Spread the mixture into a 9 by 13-inch oven-safe dish and top with the shredded cheese, then cover and freeze for up to 3 months. To heat, thaw in the fridge overnight, then place the dish in a cold oven. (You don't want to risk a glass dish shattering from a drastic temperature change.) Turn on the oven to 350°F and bake uncovered until the cheese on top is golden and the eggs in the center of the dish are cooked thoroughly, about 1 hour and 15 minutes.

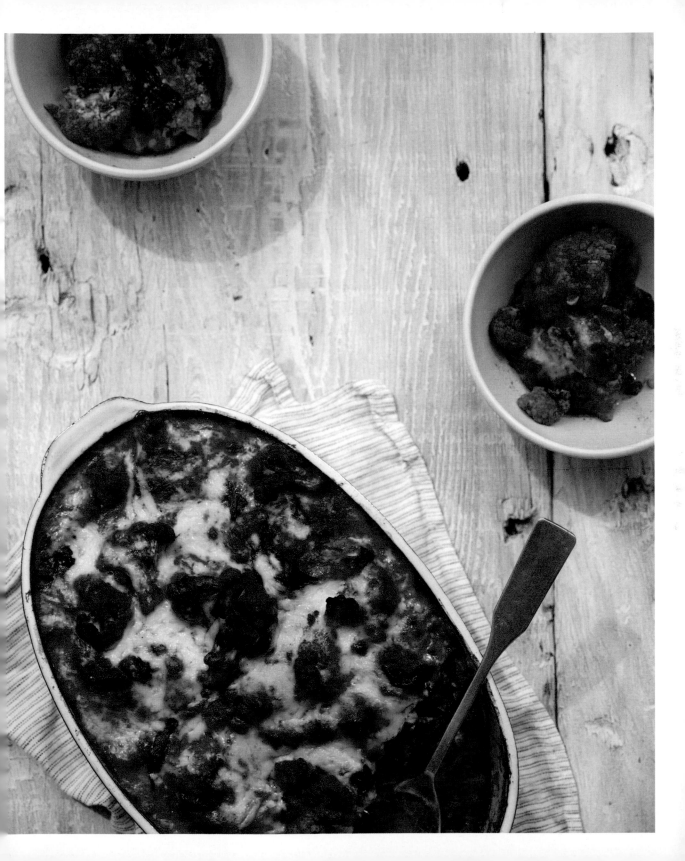

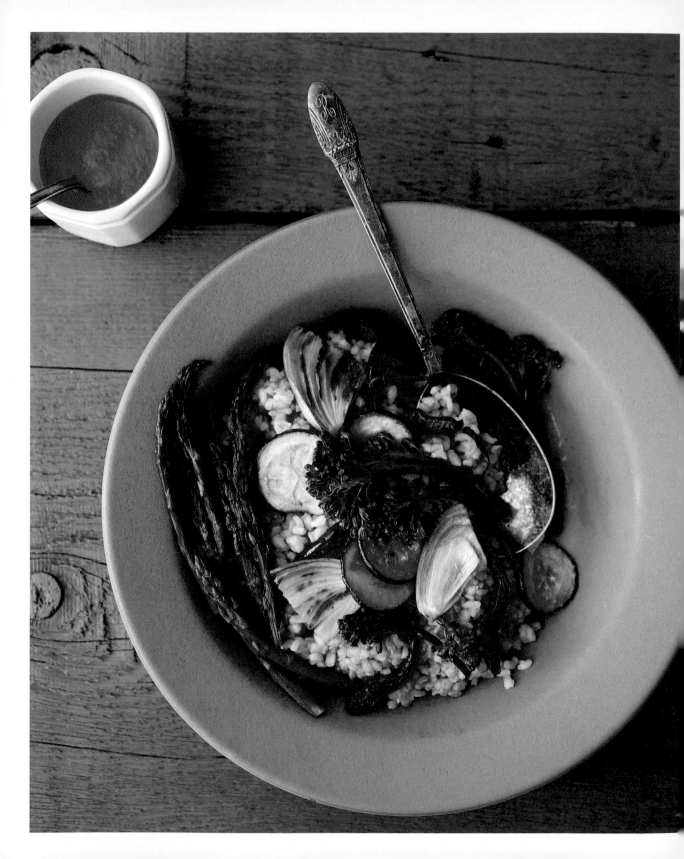

roasted vegetable rice bowls
with carrot ginger sauce

SERVES 4 | $2.89 PER SERVING

These bowls are an easy and comforting meal, perfect for a night when you don't have a lot of time for hands-on preparation. Although it does take some time for the vegetables to roast and for the rice to cook, you can be productive doing other things in your home while the veggies are unattended. This dish is completely customizable to use up any fresh produce you have on hand, so feel free to get creative with any and all of the toppings!

1 Preheat the oven to 350°F. In a single layer on two large baking sheets, arrange the broccoli, asparagus, zucchini, onion, and bell pepper. Drizzle the coconut oil over the vegetables, toss them directly in the pan to evenly coat, and sprinkle generously with salt. Roast until the vegetables are fork-tender, about 30 minutes.

2 While the vegetables are cooking, in a large saucepan, combine the rice and water and bring to a boil. Stir the rice, then cover and turn the heat to low. Simmer for 18 minutes, then remove from the heat and let the pan remain covered for 5 minutes before lifting the lid and fluffing the rice with a fork.

3 To prepare the sauce: While the rice is cooking, in a high-speed blender, combine the carrots, ginger, shallot, vinegar, honey, sesame oil, olive oil, water, and salt and blend until completely smooth. Taste and adjust any seasonings as needed.

4 Add a large scoop of rice to the bottom of each serving bowl and top generously with the roasted veggies and sauce. Serve warm. Leftover roasted vegetables and dressing can be stored separately in airtight containers in the refrigerator for up to 4 days.

MAKE IT AHEAD: For a fast freezer meal, freeze the cooked rice ahead of time in 1-cup portions, and freeze the prepared sauce in ice cube trays for easy portioning. To reheat, thaw the frozen rice and 4 to 5 sauce cubes in a skillet over medium heat, along with your favorite frozen vegetables, until heated through.

MAKE IT GRAIN-FREE: If you'd prefer to avoid rice, you can serve the roasted vegetables and sauce over a bed of cauliflower "rice" (see page 155) as a vegetable-centric alternative.

STARCH
(DF) (EF) (GF) (NF) (NS)

1 pound broccoli or broccolini, cut into florets and chopped

1 pound asparagus, tough stems removed, cut into 1-inch pieces

1 zucchini, sliced into half moons

1 red onion, thickly sliced

1 bell pepper, sliced

2 to 3 tablespoons coconut oil, melted

Fine sea salt

2 cups uncooked jasmine or basmati rice

4 cups water

CARROT GINGER SAUCE

2 medium carrots, shredded

2 tablespoons chopped fresh ginger

2 tablespoons minced shallot

2 tablespoons raw apple cider vinegar

2 tablespoons raw honey

1 tablespoon toasted sesame oil

6 tablespoons extra-virgin olive oil

¼ cup water

¾ teaspoon sea salt

speedy black bean burgers

MAKES 6 TO 8 PATTIES | $0.53 TO $0.71 PER SERVING

STARCH

(DF) (EF) (GF) (NS) (SF) (V)

1½ cups cooked black beans (see page 78) or 1 (15-ounce) can, rinsed and drained

1 cup gluten-free rolled oats

1¼ teaspoons fine sea salt

1 carrot, chopped

1 teaspoon ground cumin

1 teaspoon chili powder

½ teaspoon garlic powder

1 red bell pepper, diced

¼ red onion, diced

½ cup loosely packed fresh flat-leaf parsley, chopped

Coconut oil, for frying (optional)

6 to 8 high-quality buns or butter lettuce leaves

Your favorite toppings such as arugula, avocado, and red onion

The Quinoa & Mushroom Burgers in my first book have been a big hit with my readers, but they are a bit time-consuming to prepare, so this burger recipe is my speedy alternative! It's loaded with fiber and protein from black beans and lots of flavorful veggies, to truly earn the name of a "veggie" burger. I prefer the texture of these burgers when they are pan-fried, but I bake them more often because you can finish cooking the whole batch in less than 30 minutes. Feel free to double this recipe and freeze the extras for a quick and easy weeknight meal.

1   Preheat the oven to 350°F (if you plan to bake them) and line a baking sheet with parchment paper.

2   In the bowl of a large food processor fitted with an "S" blade, combine the beans, oats, salt, carrot, cumin, chili powder, garlic powder, bell pepper, onion, and parsley and process until a uniform mixture that sticks together is created. The mix shouldn't be supersmooth and may even resemble the texture of ground beef.

3   Use a ⅓-cup measure to scoop the burger mixture and use your hands to press into patties about ¾ inch thick, making 6 to 8 evenly sized patties. Arrange in a single layer on the prepared baking sheet.

4   To bake: Bake for 15 minutes, then gently flip with a spatula and bake for 10 minutes more. The patties are done when the outside is dry and crisp, but the inside is still tender.

5   To pan-fry: Heat a small amount of coconut oil in a cast-iron skillet over medium heat and place a patty in the center of the pan. Cook for 4 to 5 minutes, until the spatula easily slides under a crisp side, then flip and cook the other side for another 4 to 5 minutes. Repeat with the remaining patties, greasing the pan as needed to prevent sticking.

6   Serve warm with toppings on a bun or in a lettuce wrap. Store leftovers in an airtight container in the refrigerator for up to 1 week, or in the freezer for up to 6 months. (Be sure to place parchment paper between each patty to prevent sticking.) To reheat, simply heat the burgers in a skillet on both sides until the centers are warm.

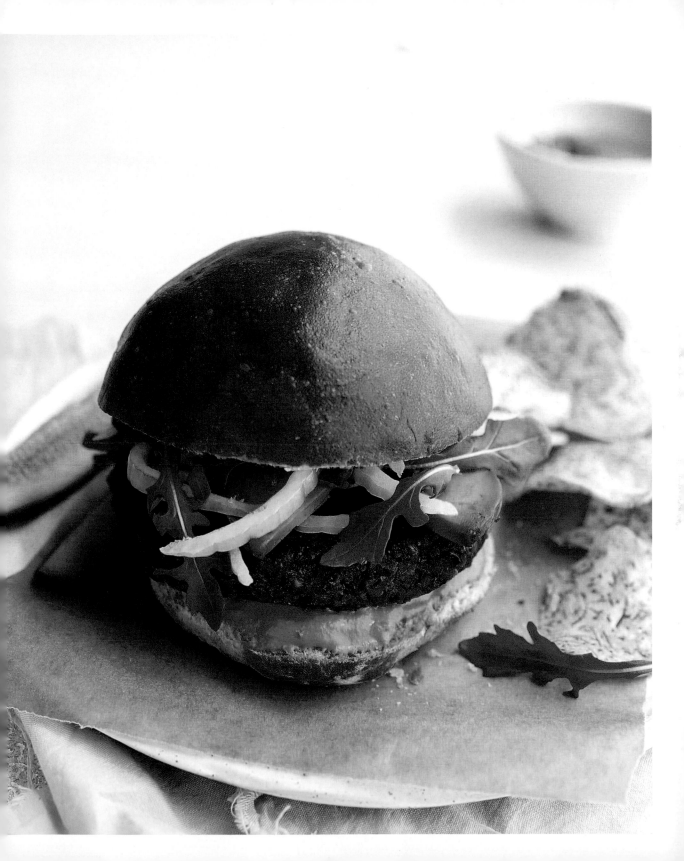

NOTE: If you'd prefer to serve these as appetizers, make 16 smaller stacks by using only one layer of each ingredient.

roasted zucchini pesto lasagna stacks

SERVES 4 (TWO PER PERSON) | $2.01 PER SERVING

These colorful vegetable stacks make a beautiful presentation for dinner guests and are easy to prepare with a lasagna-like flare. While it might sound intimidating to roast your own bell pepper, I assure you that the process is as easy as can be and the flavor makes these stacks downright irresistible. Don't be tempted to omit them. Once you get this process down, don't be surprised if this meal is requested on a weekly basis—the flavor is addictive!

1   Preheat the oven to 400°F and line two large baking sheets with parchment paper or silicone baking mats. If you like, use a vegetable peeler to peel the eggplant lengthwise leaving "stripes" of skin to help the slices hold their shape when roasted. (This technique helps you avoid biting into super-chewy skin later.) Cut the eggplant crosswise into ½-inch slices, making roughly 16 round slices. Arrange the eggplant slices in a single layer on one of the prepared baking sheets, lightly brush the tops with some of the olive oil (keep in mind the slices will absorb the oil almost instantly, so be sure to use a light touch!), and season with salt and pepper. Roast for 5 minutes.

2   Meanwhile, slice the tomatoes into ¼-inch slices, making 16 round slices, and arrange them on the second prepared baking sheet. Brush with olive oil, sprinkle with salt and pepper, and place in the oven on a separate shelf, after the eggplant has had the 5-minute head start. Roast until both vegetables are tender, about 10 minutes more (15 minutes total for the eggplant).

3   To prepare the pesto: While the veggies are roasting, in a high-speed blender or small food processor, combine the zucchini, basil, garlic, lemon juice, olive oil, and salt and blend until smooth.

4   Once the eggplant and tomatoes are tender, take the largest 8 slices of eggplant and top each with a spoonful of pesto, followed by a slice each of roasted bell pepper and tomato, and a sprinkling of cheese. Repeat the process with another layer of eggplant, pesto, bell pepper, tomato, and cheese. Return the stacks to the oven and bake until the cheese is hot and all of the veggies are heated through, about 10 minutes. Serve immediately. Store leftovers in an airtight container in the refrigerator for up to 3 days.

ANIMAL PROTEIN

1 large eggplant

2 tablespoons extra-virgin olive oil

Fine sea salt and freshly ground black pepper

2 or 3 large tomatoes

ZUCCHINI PESTO

½ zucchini, chopped

½ cup loosely packed fresh basil

2 cloves garlic

1 tablespoon freshly squeezed lemon juice

1 tablespoon extra-virgin olive oil

¼ teaspoon fine sea salt

2 Roasted Red Bell Peppers (page 190), sliced into 16 pieces

4 ounces chèvre (soft goat cheese)

vegan shepherd's pie

SERVES 4 | $1.46 PER SERVING

STARCH

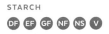

TOPPING

1½ pounds sweet potatoes or Yukon gold potatoes, peeled and chopped into 1-inch chunks

1 cup water

½ teaspoon minced fresh rosemary

FILLING

1 tablespoon coconut oil

1 yellow onion, chopped

3 carrots, chopped

2 celery stalks, chopped

2 cloves garlic, minced

8 ounces cremini mushrooms, coarsely chopped

2 teaspoons minced fresh thyme

1 teaspoon minced fresh rosemary

¾ cup dried red lentils

1 cup fresh or frozen English peas

2½ cups water

1 tablespoon raw apple cider vinegar

1 tablespoon tamari (gluten-free soy sauce)

Fine sea salt and freshly ground black pepper

This shepherd's pie is such a comforting, filling dish that it's perfect to serve as a main entrée for the holidays for your vegan friends and family. I've streamlined this recipe as much as possible, making it a quick two-pot meal. You cook everything for the filling in one pot, while the topping cooks in its own pot—you can even mash the potatoes directly in their cooking water to avoid dirtying an extra dish. If potatoes aren't your thing, feel free to use mashed cauliflower as a lower-starch alternative.

1   To prepare the topping: In a saucepan, combine the sweet potatoes, water, and rosemary, and bring to a boil over high heat. Once boiling, lower the heat to a simmer and cover the pot to let the potatoes steam until tender, about 20 minutes.

2   To prepare the filling: Meanwhile, in a separate large pot, melt the coconut oil over medium heat and sauté the onion, carrots, and celery until they start to soften, about 5 minutes. Add the garlic and sauté until fragrant, about 1 minute more. Add the mushrooms, thyme, and rosemary and sauté until the mushrooms soften, about 5 minutes. Add the lentils, peas, water, vinegar, tamari, and 1 teaspoon salt; season with pepper; and raise the heat to bring to a boil. Cover and lower the heat to a simmer, cooking until the lentils are tender, 18 to 20 minutes, then taste and adjust the seasoning. If you'd like a more gravy-like texture, use an immersion blender to puree a bit of the filling to make it creamier, while still leaving plenty of texture.

3   When the potatoes are tender, mash them directly in the cooking pot (the remaining water in the pan is the perfect amount of moisture to make the potatoes easily spreadable without using additional fat). Season with salt and pepper and then spread the mixture over the top of the cooked filling. Use the back of a spoon to smooth the sweet potato mixture evenly. Serve immediately, or bake in a 350°F oven for 30 minutes to dry out the potatoes a bit. Store the leftovers in an airtight container in the refrigerator for up to 4 days.

MAKE IT AHEAD: Use the Freezer or Slow/Pressure Cooker Method on page 15 to prepare the filling ahead of time.

NOTE: While most traditional recipes call for browning the potatoes, I prefer not to broil them because potatoes are prone to acrylamide formation, a cancer-causing agent, when browned (see page 103; the same risk does not apply when they are cooked in water.)

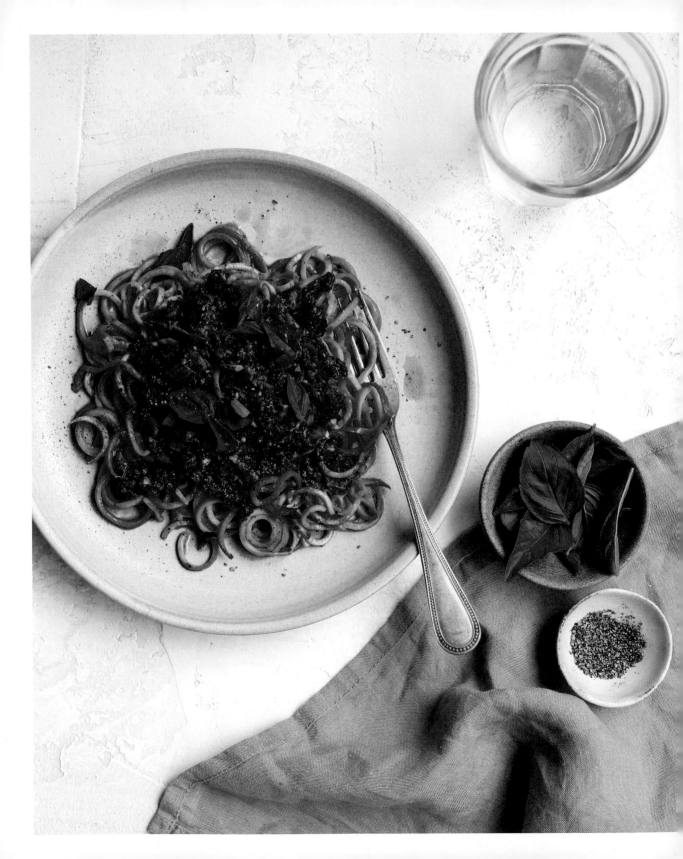

zucchini bolognese

SERVES 4 TO 6 | $ 0.82 TO $1.23 PER SERVING

This hearty sauce may soon become your go-to pasta topper. It gets its meatlike texture from vegetables that have been pulsed in a food processor, along with a few crunchy walnuts that are loaded with heart-healthy omega-3 fatty acids. When served over zucchini noodles, this is a properly combined meal that is loaded with veggies.

NUT/SEED/DRIED FRUIT

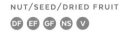

1 To prepare the sauce: In the bowl of a large food processor, combine the cauliflower and carrot and pulse until a ricelike texture is achieved. Set aside.

2 In a large pan, melt the coconut oil over medium heat and sauté the onion and bell pepper for 5 minutes. Add the garlic and cauliflower-carrot "rice" and sauté until tender and the size has reduced, another 5 to 8 minutes. Add the tomatoes, tomato paste, salt, oregano, and basil and simmer uncovered for 10 minutes to let the flavors meld. Taste and adjust the seasonings and add the maple syrup if a bit of sweetness is needed. Remove the sauce from the heat and stir in the crushed walnuts for texture.

3 While the sauce is simmering, in a separate large, deep skillet, melt the coconut oil over medium-high heat and sauté the zucchini noodles until tender, 5 to 8 minutes.

4 Serve the sauce over the zucchini noodles and top with the nutritional yeast for a "cheesy" flavor. Store leftovers in an airtight container in the refrigerator for up to 5 days.

MAKE IT AHEAD: Use the Freezer or Slow/Pressure Cooker Method on page 15.

SAUCE

8 ounces cauliflower, cut into florets

1 large carrot, cut into a few chunks

1 tablespoon coconut oil

½ yellow onion, chopped

1 red bell pepper, chopped

2 cloves garlic, minced

1 (28-ounce) box or jar chopped tomatoes (no salt or sugar added)

2 tablespoons tomato paste

1 teaspoon fine sea salt

1 teaspoon dried oregano

1 teaspoon dried basil

1 teaspoon maple syrup (optional)

½ cup crushed walnuts

1 teaspoon coconut oil

4 medium zucchini, spiralized into "noodles"

Dash of nutritional yeast (optional)

enchilada-stuffed zucchini boats

SERVES 4 | $2.69 PER SERVING

ANIMAL PROTEIN

FILLING

1 tablespoon butter
or coconut oil

1 red onion, chopped

1 red bell pepper,
chopped

1 jalapeño chile, seeded
and chopped

2 cloves garlic, minced

1 pound tomatoes,
chopped

½ teaspoon fine
sea salt

1 teaspoon ground
cumin

1 teaspoon chili powder

4 large zucchini

3 ounces goat cheddar,
shredded

These zucchini boats are an easier and healthier way to enjoy your favorite enchilada flavors more often. Instead of making a complicated mock tortilla, this flavorful filling is stuffed into juicy zucchini halves and roasted with a topping of melted cheese for an enchilada-like experience, without any extra effort. I think you'll find that this version is just as satisfying, even without the greasy meat or starchy tortillas!

1   Preheat the oven to 400°F and line a large baking sheet with parchment paper.

2   To prepare the filling: In a large skillet, melt the butter over medium heat and sauté the onion, bell pepper, and jalapeño until tender, about 10 minutes. Add the garlic, tomatoes, salt, cumin, and chili powder and sauté until the tomatoes are tender and much of their moisture has been released, another 8 to 10 minutes.

3   While the filling is cooking, slice the zucchini in half lengthwise (cut off the hard top) and use a teaspoon to scoop out the soft centers. (Add the zucchini flesh to the cooked vegetables if you like, too!) Be sure to leave enough of the zucchini flesh so that the bottoms of the zucchini boats are sturdy enough to hold the filling—you don't want to scrape them too thin. Arrange the zucchini shells cut-side up on the prepared baking sheet and fill each one with the cooked tomato mixture. Top each "boat" with the cheese.

4   Bake the boats until the zucchini is tender and the cheese is bubbly, about 20 minutes. Serve immediately.

MAKE IT AHEAD: Refrigerate the uncooked, filled zucchini, covered, for up to 3 days. To heat, place the dish in a cold oven. Turn on the oven to 350°F and bake until the cheese is golden and the zucchini are fork-tender, about 40 minutes. As an alternative, the filling also freezes well, so you can make it ahead of time, freeze for up to 3 months, and then thaw it overnight in the refrigerator the day before you plan on serving it. Simply add the thawed filling to the zucchini halves and bake as directed.

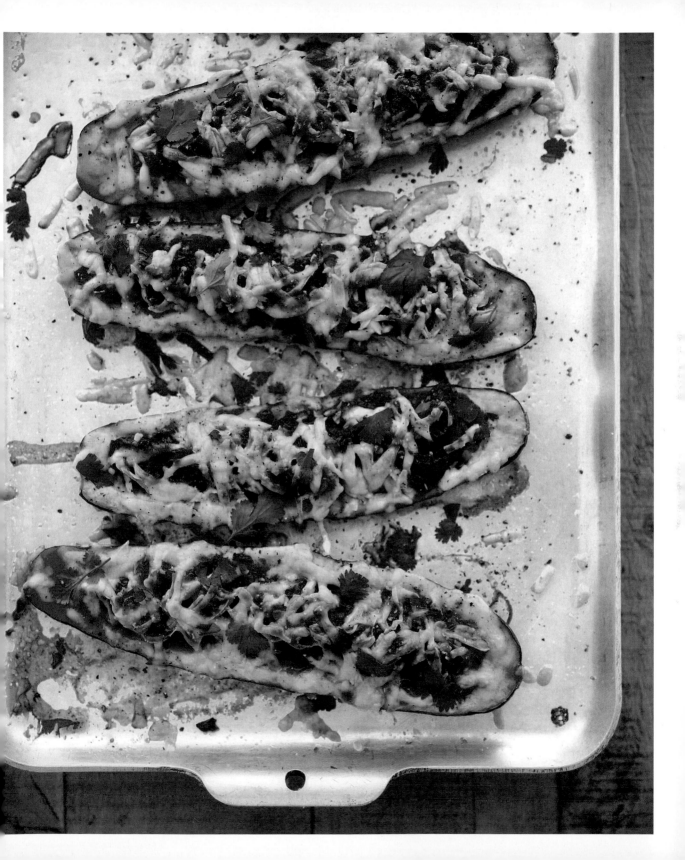

"cheesy" broccoli quinoa casserole

SERVES 4 | $1.73 PER SERVING

STARCH

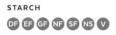

1 cup quinoa, rinsed and drained

2½ cups water

1 teaspoon coconut oil

½ yellow onion, chopped

5 cups broccoli florets

"CHEESE" SAUCE

1 cup mashed sweet potato

1½ cups water

1 tablespoon freshly squeezed lemon juice

¼ cup nutritional yeast

2 teaspoons fine sea salt

1 teaspoon onion powder

½ teaspoon chili powder

This creamy casserole reminds me of a favorite childhood dish that my mom simply called broccoli and rice. In this version, I've replaced the rice with quinoa, which is a complete source of protein, and paired it with a creamy "cheese" sauce made from sweet potatoes and nutritional yeast. Nutritional yeast is a great source of minerals, including magnesium and zinc, and is rich in B vitamins; its cheeselike flavor works well in many vegan dishes. When served together with a hefty dose of broccoli, this dish is everything a casserole should be—warm, filling, and comforting!

1 Preheat the oven to 350°F.

2 In a small saucepan, bring the quinoa and 2 cups of the water to a boil over high heat, then cover, turn the heat to low, and cook for 15 minutes, until the quinoa is tender and the moisture has been absorbed. Fluff with a fork and set aside.

3 Meanwhile, in a large Dutch oven, melt the coconut oil over medium heat and sauté the onion until it starts to soften, about 5 minutes. Add the broccoli and remaining ½ cup water (which should immediately start steaming when it hits the pan), to prevent sticking. Cover the pan and allow to steam for about 10 minutes, or until the broccoli is fork-tender.

4 To prepare the sauce: In a high-speed blender, combine the sweet potato, water, lemon juice, nutritional yeast, salt, onion powder, and chili powder and blend until completely smooth and creamy.

5 Once the broccoli is tender, add the cooked quinoa to the Dutch oven and then the sauce. Stir to mix well. Taste and adjust any seasonings. Serve warm. Store leftovers in an airtight container in the refrigerator for up to 5 days.

MAKE IT AHEAD: This "cheese" sauce freezes well, so make it ahead of time and freeze it in ice-cube trays for up to 3 months for easy reheating. Simply stir the cubes into the hot quinoa and broccoli until thoroughly heated, and serve warm.

comforting vegetable korma

SERVES 2 | $3.95 PER SERVING

Vegetable korma, featuring tender assorted vegetables served in a mildly spiced creamy sauce, is my very favorite dish to order at Indian restaurants. If you're like me and are slightly intimidated by making Indian food at home, prepared spice blends like garam masala and curry powder make the process much easier, since they're available in most grocery stores. In this particular version, I used mild vegetables like cauliflower, potatoes, and carrots because they soak up the flavors of the sauce so well, but you can use any veggies you like, except for sweet potatoes, which simply don't work well with this flavor profile, if you ask me. Serve this creamy vegetable dish over rice to soak up any extra sauce—you won't want to waste a bite!

1   In a large sauce pot, melt the coconut oil over medium-high heat and sauté the onion until tender, about 10 minutes. Add the garlic, ginger, garam masala, and curry powder and sauté until fragrant, another 1 or 2 minutes.

2   Add the coconut milk, tomato puree, salt, and maple syrup and stir well to dissolve the spices.

3   Add the cauliflower, potatoes, carrots, and peas to the pot and bring the liquid to a boil. Lower the heat to a simmer and then cover with a lid to let the vegetables cook until tender, 15 to 20 minutes. Taste and adjust any seasonings. Serve warm over a bed of rice, garnished with cilantro. Store leftovers in an airtight container in the refrigerator for up to 4 days.

MAKE IT AHEAD: Use the Freezer or Slow/Pressure Cooker Method on page 15.

STARCH

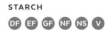

1 tablespoon
coconut oil

1 small yellow onion

3 cloves garlic

1-inch knob of fresh
ginger, peeled and
minced

2 teaspoons garam
masala

1 teaspoon curry
powder

1 (15-ounce) can full-fat
coconut milk

½ cup tomato puree
(strained tomatoes)

1½ teaspoons fine
sea salt

1 tablespoon
maple syrup

1 small head of
cauliflower, cut into
florets

1 pound Yukon gold
potatoes, cut into
1-inch chunks

2 carrots, diced

1 cup fresh or
frozen peas

Cooked rice or
cauliflower rice (see
page 155), for serving

Fresh cilantro, for
garnish

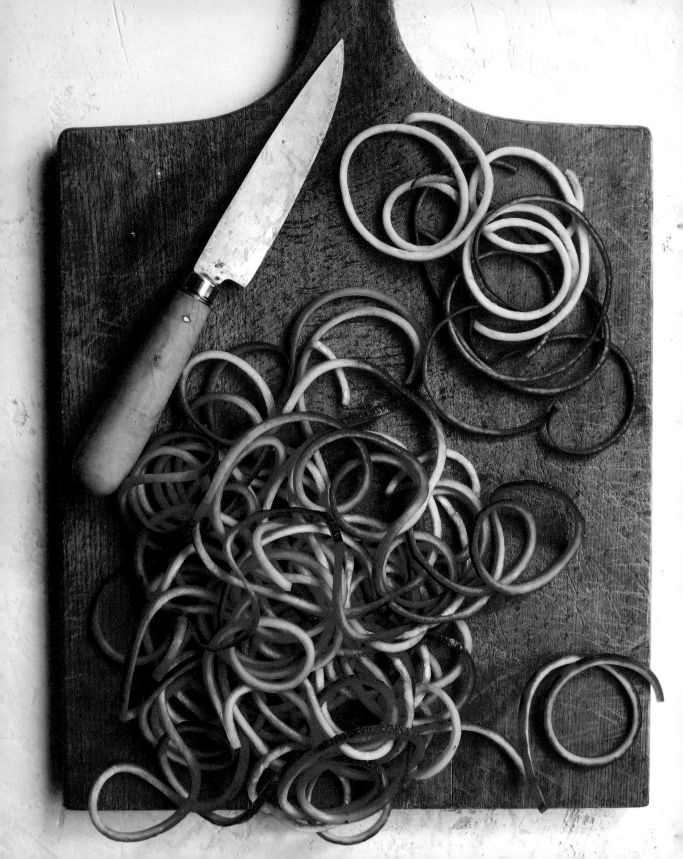

7 SKILLETS & STIR-FRIES

butternut stuffing

SERVES 4 | $1.66 PER SERVING

STARCH

1 tablespoon
coconut oil

1 large yellow onion,
chopped

3 celery stalks, chopped

2 cloves garlic, minced

8 ounces mushrooms,
chopped

2 pounds butternut
squash, peeled and
cubed

3 tablespoons chopped
fresh sage

1 tablespoon chopped
fresh thyme

2 teaspoons fine
sea salt

½ cup dried cranberries
or raisins (optional)

½ cup chopped pecans
(optional)

Stuffing is one of my family's favorite comfort food dishes, to the point that my dad requests it year-round. This recipe is my solution—it's healthy enough to eat on a daily basis but has all of the holiday flavors you crave. I like to add pecans and cranberries for a variety of texture and flavors, which technically is not properly combined, but this dish is so clean that it should still digest smoothly. I hope you'll enjoy it all year long!

1   In a large Dutch oven, melt the coconut oil over medium-high heat and sauté the onion and celery until tender, about 8 minutes. Add the mushrooms and garlic and cook for another 5 minutes, until they are tender as well.

2   While the vegetables are cooking, place the butternut squash in a food processor fitted with an "S" blade and process until the squash is ricelike in texture. (This should take 10 to 20 seconds.)

3   Add the butternut "rice" to the cooked vegetables, along with the sage, thyme, and salt. Sauté until the squash is tender, 8 to 10 minutes.

4   Remove the pan from the heat and stir in the cranberries and pecans. Serve warm. Store leftovers in an airtight container in the refrigerator for up to 4 days.

MISS THE MEAT? This dish is properly combined if you replace the butternut squash with cauliflower or carrot "rice." When this recipe is made with a low-starch vegetable, you can add meat if you like—such as leftover turkey—for a meal that truly tastes like Thanksgiving in a bowl.

MAKE IT AHEAD: Combine all of the ingredients, except for the dried fruit and pecans, in a 1-gallon freezer-safe container and freeze for up to 6 months. To heat, thaw in the refrigerator overnight, then transfer the vegetables to a 9 by 13-inch oven-safe dish. Place the dish in a cold oven. Turn on the oven to 350°F and bake until the vegetables are piping hot and golden, about 60 minutes. Stir in the dried cranberries and pecans, and serve warm.

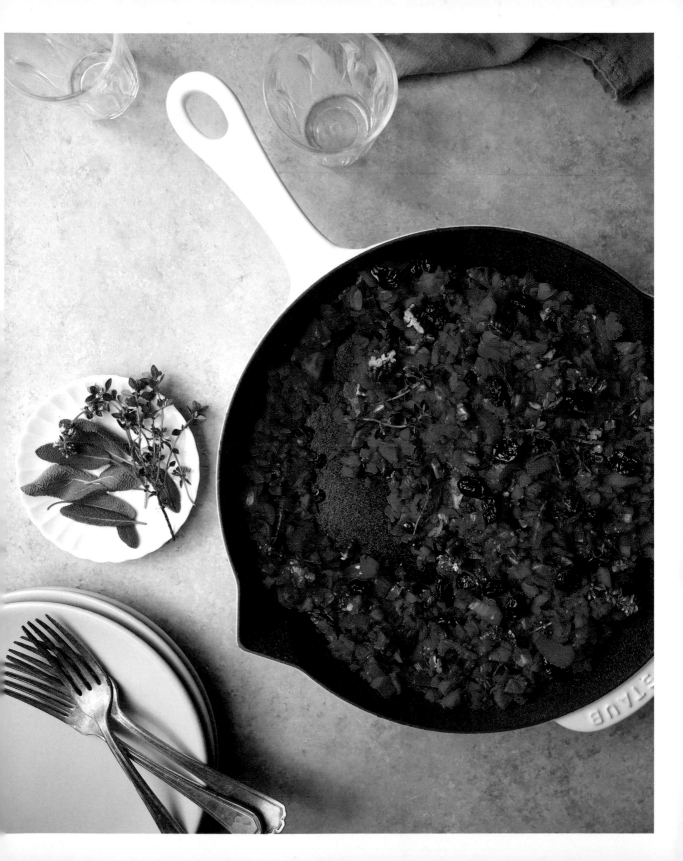

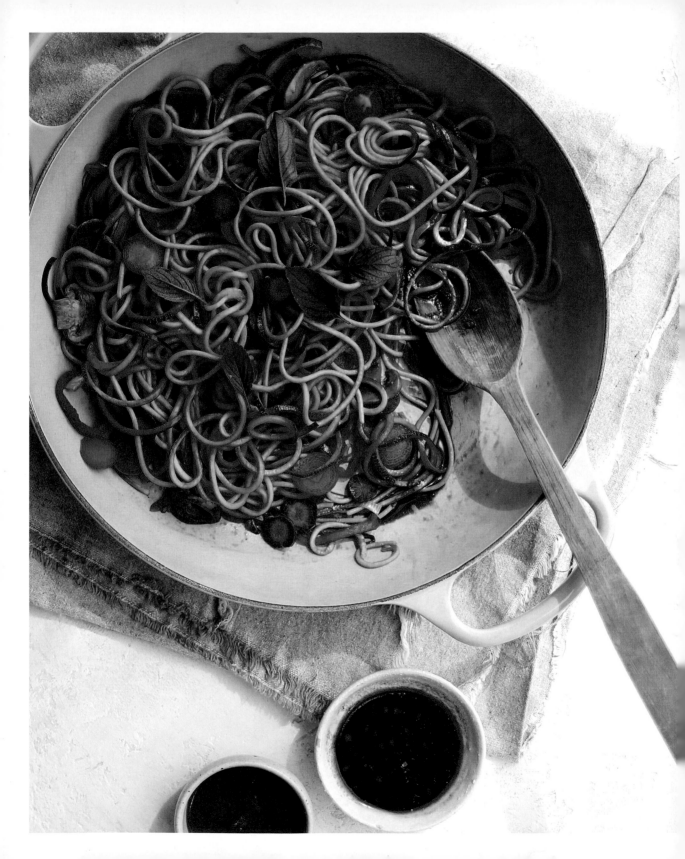

rainbow lo mein

SERVES 2 (AS A MEAL) | $3.32 PER SERVING

While some people might find it easy to replace regular pasta with zucchini "noodles," that's not always the case for everyone—even for my own family members. This lo mein dish is my solution, since it takes a fifty-fifty approach, using half pasta and half zucchini noodles for a more vegetable-centric dish that is still as satisfying as the traditional version. Feel free to add any vegetables you have on hand to make this recipe your own.

STARCH

4 ounces brown rice spaghetti noodles

1 Prepare the spaghetti according to the package directions.

2 To prepare the sauce: In a small bowl, whisk together the tamari, honey, ginger, Sriracha, and sesame oil and set aside.

3 Use a spiralizer to turn the zucchini into spaghetti-like noodles or use a vegetable peeler to create long, thin zucchini ribbons, then set them aside.

4 While the spaghetti is cooking, in a large Dutch oven, melt the coconut oil over medium heat and sauté the onion and bell pepper until tender, about 10 minutes. Add the carrots, zucchini, and mushrooms, along with the reserved sauce, and sauté until tender, another 5 to 8 minutes.

5 Add the pasta and toss well to coat in the sauce. Adjust any seasonings, adding an extra splash of tamari or Sriracha, if desired. Once everything is tender and heated through, the dish is ready to serve. Store leftovers in an airtight container in the refrigerator for up to 3 days.

SAUCE

¼ cup tamari (gluten-free soy sauce)

2 teaspoons honey

2 teaspoons minced fresh ginger

1 teaspoon Sriracha

1 teaspoon toasted sesame oil

1 (8-ounce) zucchini

1 tablespoon coconut oil

1 red onion, thinly sliced

1 red bell pepper, thinly sliced

2 large carrots, julienned

8 ounces mushrooms, sliced

MAKE IT GRAIN-FREE: If you'd prefer to skip the pasta altogether, simply replace the spaghetti with two additional spiralized zucchini for a completely vegetable-based dish. In this case, you can add meat to it for a properly combined meal.

MAKE IT AHEAD: This dish is delicious served hot or cold, so feel free to make it up to 3 days in advance and store it in an airtight container in the fridge until ready to serve. Serve cold, or reheat in a large Dutch oven over medium heat, stirring until piping hot, 5 to 8 minutes. (Add a splash of water to prevent sticking, if needed.)

zucchini "pasta" primavera

SERVES 2 | $4.20 PER SERVING

ANIMAL PROTEIN

2 large zucchini

1 tablespoon coconut oil or butter

1 red onion, thinly sliced

1 carrot, julienned

1 red bell pepper, chopped

1 pound asparagus, tough stems removed, chopped (see Note)

2 cloves garlic, minced

1 pint cherry tomatoes, sliced in half

½ teaspoon fine sea salt

1 teaspoon dried basil

1 teaspoon dried oregano

6 tablespoons grated Pecorino Romano cheese

Pinch of red pepper flakes (optional)

Pasta primavera is a popular dish featuring lightly sautéed vegetables, so I decided to take it a step further by making it entirely vegetable-based using zucchini "noodles" as the pasta. Zucchini is surprisingly satisfying as a pasta alternative, and when it is tossed with other flavorful spring vegetables, herbs, and a touch of cheese, no one will miss the traditional version at all.

1   Using a spiralizer, turn the zucchini into spaghetti-like noodles or use a vegetable peeler to create long, thin zucchini ribbons, then set them aside.

2   In a large pot, melt the coconut oil over medium heat and sauté the onion and carrot for 5 minutes. Add the bell pepper and asparagus and sauté until all the veggies are tender, about 8 minutes more. Add the garlic and sauté until fragrant, about 1 minute. Add the zucchini noodles, tomatoes, salt, basil, oregano, and red pepper flakes, and sauté until the zucchini is tender, 5 to 8 minutes.

3   Remove the pot from the heat. Sprinkle the cheese over the top and adjust the seasoning, if needed. Serve warm. Store leftovers in an airtight container in the refrigerator for up to 3 days.

MISS THE MEAT? You are welcome to add your favorite high-quality meat toppings to this stir-fry for a properly combined dish. Just add it in while cooking the peppers and asparagus in step 2 and drain off any juices.

NOTE: When asparagus isn't in season, feel free to use chopped broccoli as a substitute.

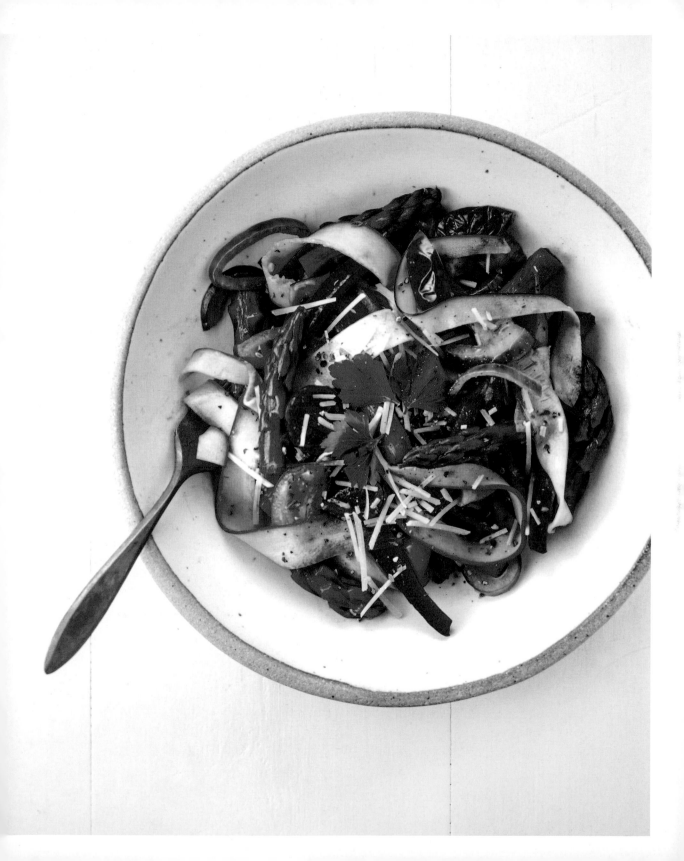

one-pot quinoa fried rice

SERVES 4 | $2.30 PER SERVING

30-MINUTE RECIPE
KID-FRIENDLY

STARCH

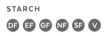

1 tablespoon
coconut oil

1 yellow onion, chopped

3 carrots, chopped

3 celery stalks, chopped

1-inch knob of fresh
ginger, peeled and
minced

2 cloves garlic, minced

8 ounces mushrooms,
chopped

1 small head of broccoli,
chopped

1 zucchini, chopped

¼ cup tamari (gluten-
free soy sauce)

1 cup quinoa, rinsed
and drained

2 cups water

Fine sea salt

Sriracha (optional)

This recipe is for those who love the flavor of fried rice but would prefer to avoid greasy takeout. Quinoa is a complete source of protein, containing all of the essential amino acids we need, and it cooks in just 15 minutes. In this case, it actually cooks in the same pot as all of the veggies and sauce, so everything is ready in no time!

1   In a large Dutch oven or pot, melt the coconut oil over medium heat and sauté the onion, carrots, and celery until tender, about 10 minutes. Add the ginger and garlic and sauté until fragrant, about 1 minute more.

2   Add the mushrooms, broccoli, zucchini, and tamari and toss well to coat the veggies in the sauce. Add the quinoa and water and bring everything to a boil. Cover and simmer until the quinoa and broccoli are tender, about 15 minutes.

3   Remove the lid and stir well to ensure all of the liquid has been absorbed. Season with salt and add a squeeze of Sriracha if you'd like it to be on the spicier side. Serve warm. Store leftovers in an airtight container in the refrigerator for up to 5 days.

NOTE: As written, the vegetables in this recipe are very tender, which is how my family prefers them. If you would like more of a bite to your broccoli, wait to add it until the quinoa has only 10 minutes left to cook.

pizza stir-fry

SERVES 2 TO 4 | $0.97 TO $1.94 PER SERVING

30-MINUTE RECIPE

This recipe was created out of necessity one night, when I was trying to stay on budget by using the leftover ingredients we had on hand. The result was so unbelievably delicious that it has become a weekly staple. We are always looking for an excuse to eat more pizzalike dishes, so I hope you enjoy it just as much as we do.

1   In a large pot, melt the coconut oil over medium heat and sauté the onion and both bell peppers until tender, about 8 minutes.

2   Add the kale, cabbage, tomato paste, salt, and oregano, and sauté until the greens begin to wilt. Add the water to help prevent sticking, and cover the pot to let the veggies cook until tender, 8 to 10 minutes.

3   Remove the lid and stir, then raise the heat to simmer off any excess liquid. Taste and adjust any seasonings. Serve warm, with a sprinkling of feta over the top. Store leftovers in an airtight container in the refrigerator for up to 4 days.

NOTE: You can use Pizza Sauce (page 186) instead of tomato paste if you like. Replace the tomato paste with ¾ to 1 cup Pizza Sauce, to taste.

MISS THE MEAT? You are welcome to add your favorite high-quality meat toppings to this pizza stir-fry for a properly combined dish. Just add it in while cooking the onion and bell peppers in step 1 and drain off any juices.

MAKE IT VEGAN: Omit the cheese and add a sprinkling of nutritional yeast instead.

ANIMAL PROTEIN

1 teaspoon coconut oil or butter

1 yellow onion, chopped

1 green bell pepper, chopped

1 red bell pepper, chopped

2 cups shredded kale

3 pounds cabbage, shredded

1 (7-ounce) jar tomato paste (no salt added)

1 teaspoon fine sea salt

2 teaspoons dried oregano

¼ cup water, or as needed

4 ounces goat feta cheese, crumbled (optional)

singapore sweet potato noodles

SERVES 2 | $2.94 PER SERVING

STARCH

2 medium sweet
potatoes, peeled

SAUCE

2 teaspoons sesame oil

1 tablespoon minced
fresh ginger

1 clove garlic, minced

¼ cup tamari (gluten-
free soy sauce)

1 tablespoon raw apple
cider vinegar

1 tablespoon maple
syrup (optional)

2 to 3 teaspoons
curry powder

1 teaspoon coconut oil

1 red bell pepper,
chopped

3 cups mung bean
sprouts or shredded
cabbage (about
12 ounces)

6 green onions, white
and light green parts,
thinly sliced

1 cup fresh or frozen
peas

Fresh cilantro, for
garnish

This curried noodle dish is popular in Asian-style restaurants because it's an easy way for chefs to use up any veggies they have on hand. You can essentially add any fresh produce you like and taste as you go, so you always wind up with a perfectly seasoned dish that you will love. If you can find mung bean sprouts in your grocer's refrigerated section, they add a lovely crunch and noodlelike texture to this dish; shredded cabbage also makes an enjoyable alternative.

1 Using a spiralizer, turn the sweet potatoes into spaghetti-like noodles or use a vegetable peeler to create long, thin ribbons, then set them aside.

2 To prepare the sauce: In a small bowl, whisk together the sesame oil, ginger, garlic, tamari, vinegar, maple syrup, and 2 teaspoons of the curry powder, then set aside.

3 In a large Dutch oven, melt the coconut oil over medium heat and sauté the bell pepper until it starts to soften, about 5 minutes. Add the bean sprouts and reserved sauce and sauté until the vegetables shrink in size, about 5 minutes more. Add the sweet potato noodles, green onions, and peas and toss well to combine. Partially cover the pot and cook until the potatoes are tender, 8 to 10 minutes.

4 Taste and adjust the seasonings, adding more curry powder, if desired. Serve warm, garnished with cilantro. Store leftovers in an airtight container in the refrigerator for up to 3 days.

MAKE IT AHEAD: Sweet potatoes freeze very well, so you can make the raw noodles ahead of time, freeze for up to 3 months, and pull out of the freezer as needed. Thaw them directly in the Dutch oven while you prepare this recipe, keeping in mind that the dish may need a few minutes longer to cook.

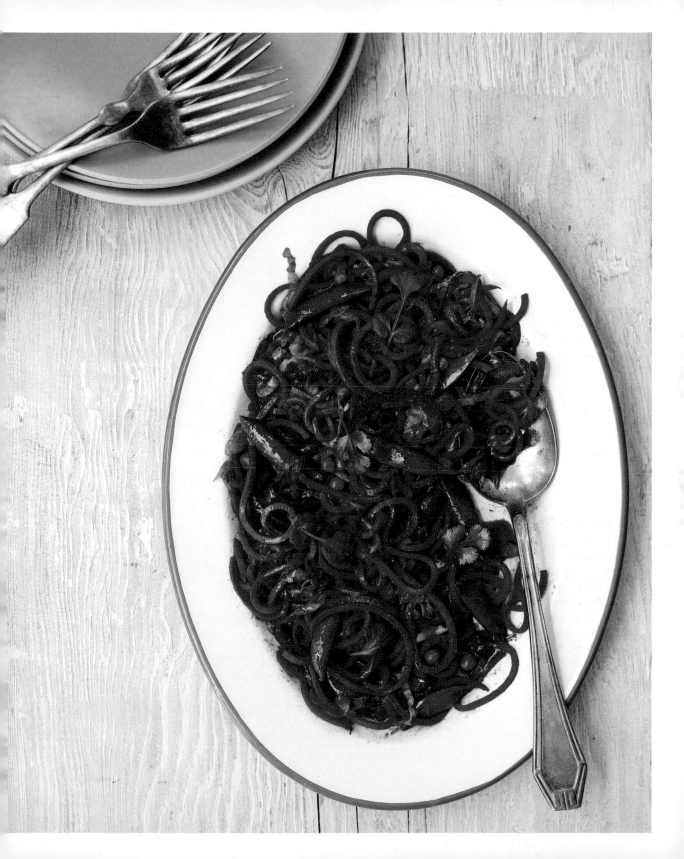

pad see ew

SERVES 2 | $3.60 PER SERVING

ANIMAL PROTEIN

(DF) (GF) (NF)

3 or 4 parsnips

1 tablespoon coconut oil

3 cloves garlic, minced

3 cups chopped broccoli florets

¼ cup water, or as needed

¼ cup tamari (gluten-free soy sauce)

1½ tablespoons maple syrup

4 eggs

Pad see ew is my husband's favorite Thai dish, featuring egg noodles tossed with eggs, broccoli, and a sweet soy sauce. It's so simple yet so tasty! I've adapted this popular dish to be almost entirely vegetable-based, using parsnip "noodles" for a tasty and nutrient-rich alternative. When cooked in the sweet soy sauce and tossed with protein-rich eggs and broccoli, it tastes surprisingly like the original. If parsnips are difficult to locate, use another vegetable, such as carrots or zucchini squash, to make your "noodles."

1   Lay each parsnip on a flat surface and, using a Y-shaped vegetable peeler, peel into ribbonlike "noodles" until you reach the center of the vegetable. Flip them and repeat the same method on the other side until you can't peel anymore. Set the noodles aside.

2   In a 5.5-quart or larger Dutch oven, melt the coconut oil over medium heat and sauté the garlic until fragrant, about 1 minute. Add the broccoli and sauté for another 5 minutes, adding the water if needed to prevent the garlic from sticking to the bottom of the pot. Add the parsnip noodles, tamari, and maple syrup and toss well to coat. (Your pan might be very full at this point until the noodles cook down.) Cover and let the noodles cook until they shrink in size, about 5 minutes, then remove the lid and continue stirring and cooking until the noodles are tender and the liquid at the bottom of the pan has evaporated.

3   Push the cooked veggies to one side of the pan and crack the eggs into the other side. Scramble them well, toss with the rest of the vegetables, then taste and adjust any seasoning. Serve warm. Store leftovers in an airtight container in the refrigerator for up to 3 days.

MISS THE MEAT? You are welcome to add your favorite high-quality meat to this properly combined dish. Simply add it in while sautéeing the broccoli in step 2 to make sure it gets thoroughly cooked by the time your vegetable noodles are tender. Drain off any juices.

cauliflower jambalaya

SERVES 4 | $2.03 PER SERVING

Cauliflower fried "rice" has become a staple in my family's diet, so I wanted to come up with a new way to spice it up—and this Creole-style dish has been declared a new favorite! As written, the dish is purely vegetable-based, but you can bulk it up as a main course by adding more protein. My husband prefers meat, but vegetarians can use black beans or chickpeas for an extra boost of protein and fiber.

NEUTRAL

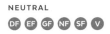

1 tablespoon coconut oil

1 yellow onion, chopped

1 green bell pepper, chopped

4 celery stalks, chopped

3 cloves garlic, minced

½ jalapeño chile, seeded and finely chopped

2 large tomatoes, chopped

1½ teaspoons paprika

1 teaspoon garlic powder

¼ teaspoon cayenne pepper

½ teaspoon dried oregano

1 head of cauliflower (about 2 pounds), cut into florets

1½ to 2 teaspoons fine sea salt

¼ cup tomato paste

1 teaspoon tamari (gluten-free soy sauce)

1 (15-ounce) can black beans or chickpeas, rinsed and drained (optional)

1   In a large 5.5-quart Dutch oven, melt the coconut oil over medium heat and sauté the onion, bell pepper, and celery until they start to soften, about 5 minutes. Add the garlic, jalapeño, tomatoes, paprika, garlic powder, cayenne, and oregano and sauté until the tomatoes release their juices and cook down, about 5 minutes more.

2   While the veggies are cooking, pulse the cauliflower florets in a food processor until a ricelike texture is achieved. Add the cauliflower rice to the sautéed vegetables, along with the salt, tomato paste and tamari and sauté until tender, about 10 minutes more. Add the beans. Stir occasionally while cooking to prevent sticking.

3   Once all of the vegetables are tender and any added protein is cooked thoroughly, taste and adjust the seasonings. Serve warm. Store leftovers in an airtight container in the refrigerator for up to 3 days.

MISS THE MEAT? Add your favorite high-quality meat, such as chicken or nitrate-free sausage, to this properly combined dish by sautéeing it with the spices in step 1.

Cauliflower Rice

Cauliflower "rice" is a versatile side dish that can be served with any number of entrées as a grain-free alternative to rice. As an easy side dish, simply pulse raw cauliflower florets in a food processor until a ricelike texture is achieved, then sauté in a deep skillet with coconut oil, a splash of water, and salt until tender, 10 to 15 minutes.

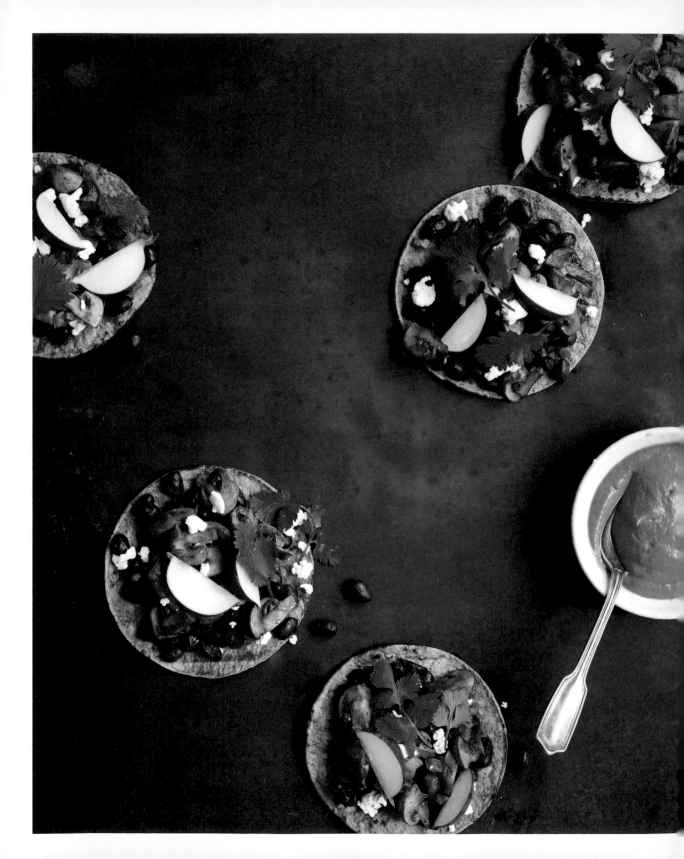

mushroom & black bean tacos
with avocado crema

MAKES 8 TACOS | $0.75 PER TACO

These tacos are a satisfying alternative for meat eaters who want to include more plant-based meals in their routine. The flavor of this hearty filling reminds me of the drive-thru tacos I ate too often in college, but this version is loaded with fiber and B vitamins, thanks to the addition of meaty mushrooms. This filling can be served in your favorite organic taco shells or in butter lettuce cups for a naturally gluten-free option. They make a great burrito filling, too!

1   To prepare the filling: In a 3.5-quart or larger Dutch oven, melt the coconut oil over medium heat and sauté the onion until translucent, about 8 minutes. Add the mushrooms and garlic and continue to sauté until the mushrooms release their liquid, about 8 minutes more.

2   Add ½ teaspoon salt, the cumin, chili powder, paprika, and black beans and sauté until heated through. Add the cayenne, then taste and adjust any seasonings. (I typically use ¾ teaspoon salt total.) Lower the heat to keep the filling warm while you prepare the crema.

3   To prepare the crema: In a high-speed blender or mini food processor, combine the avocado, lime juice, salt, cumin, honey, cilantro, garlic, and 1 tablespoon water and blend until smooth. Add additional water, if needed, to facilitate blending, then taste and adjust any seasonings.

4   Fill each tortilla generously with the filling, then top with garnishes and a spoonful of the crema. Serve warm. Store any leftover filling and crema in separate airtight containers in the refrigerator for up to 3 days. To help prevent the crema from browning, press a piece of parchment paper to the top surface and remove it right before serving again, scraping away any brown spots that might have developed.

STARCH

DF EF GF NF NS V

FILLING

1 tablespoon coconut oil

1 red onion, diced

8 ounces mushrooms, coarsely chopped

2 cloves garlic, minced

Fine sea salt

1 teaspoon ground cumin

½ teaspoon chili powder

½ teaspoon paprika

1½ cups cooked black beans (see page 78) or 1 (15-ounce) can, rinsed and drained

⅛ teaspoon cayenne pepper (optional)

AVOCADO CREMA

1 ripe Hass avocado

2 tablespoons freshly squeezed lime juice

¼ teaspoon fine sea salt

½ teaspoon ground cumin

1 teaspoon raw honey

¼ cup fresh cilantro

1 clove garlic, minced

8 gluten-free tortillas or butter lettuce leaves

Radishes and cilantro, to garnish (optional)

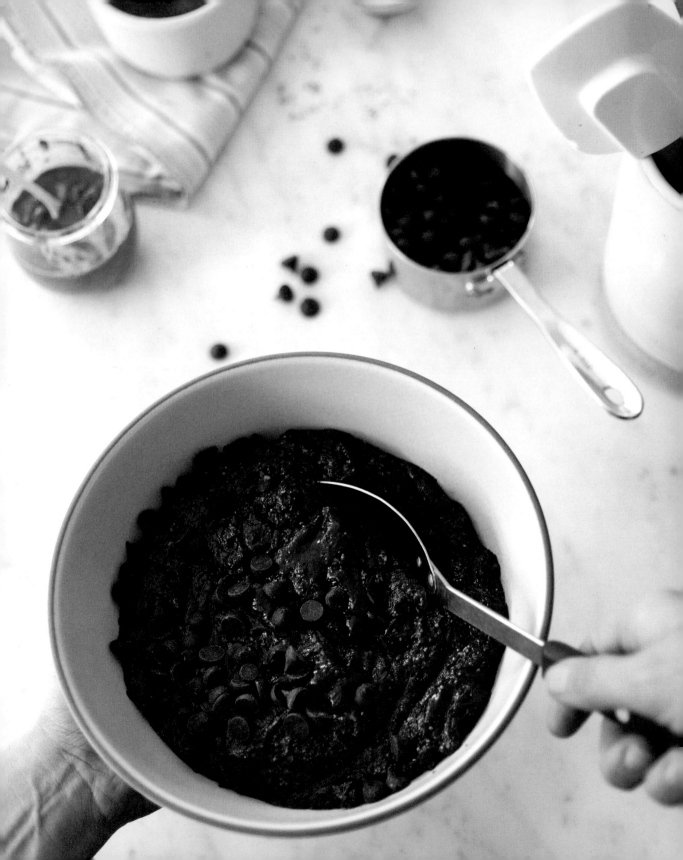

8 SWEET TREATS

chewy vegan ginger cookies

MAKES 12 COOKIES | $0.40 PER COOKIE

NUT/SEED/DRIED FRUIT

(DF) (EF) (GF) (NS) (V)

1½ cups almond flour

2 tablespoons coconut oil, melted

¼ cup maple syrup

1 tablespoon blackstrap molasses

2 teaspoons ground ginger

⅛ teaspoon fine sea salt

¼ teaspoon baking soda

These soft and chewy ginger cookies (pictured on page vi, opposite the contents) are a holiday favorite, but they are also addictive enough to enjoy year-round. The combination of molasses and ginger gives these cookies their signature flavor, but both of these ingredients are packed with health benefits, too! Blackstrap molasses is loaded with essential minerals like iron and calcium, and ginger has powerful antioxidant and anti-inflammatory properties[1] and may help to lower blood sugar levels.[2] Keep a stash of these treats in your freezer to enjoy any time of the year.

1   Preheat the oven to 250°F and line a large baking sheet with parchment paper. In a large bowl, combine the almond flour, coconut oil, maple syrup, molasses, ginger, salt, and baking soda and stir well to create a sticky batter.

2   Using a tablespoon as a scoop, drop the batter onto the prepared baking sheet, spacing the mounds about 2 inches apart. Wet your hands with water (to prevent them from sticking to the batter) and gently flatten the mounds into your desired cookie shape, about ½ inch thick.

3   Bake for 30 minutes, then remove the cookies from the oven and allow to cool completely. The edges should look dry, but the cookies will be very soft to the touch until they cool completely. Once cool, the cookies should have a dry texture on the outside and be soft and chewy inside.

4   For the best texture, store the cookies in the freezer, where they will become firm and crisp and will quickly thaw to their soft and chewy state again, for up to 6 months. (We have been known to eat them directly from the freezer, too!) When stored in an airtight container at room temperature, the cookies will become very soft and stick together, and will be more prone to mold, so don't leave them out for more than 48 hours.

NOTE: Baking these almond-based cookies at a low temperature keeps their delicate oils intact and helps prevent the formation of acrylamide, a harmful carcinogen (see page 103).

coconut oatmeal raisin cookies

MAKES ABOUT 16 COOKIES | $0.32 PER COOKIE

Trying to create a cookie that is nut-free, gluten-free, and vegan can be quite the challenge, but these allergy-friendly options fit the bill. They have a slightly chewy texture, thanks to the addition of shredded coconut, which adds bulk without drying out the cookies the way rolled oats can. Paired with low-glycemic coconut sugar and ground chia seeds that create a vegan egglike substitute, these cookies pack plenty of fiber to help you avoid a sugar crash later.

1   Preheat the oven to 350°F and line a baking sheet with parchment paper. In a small bowl, combine the ground chia seeds and water, then stir and set aside while you mix the rest of the ingredients.

2   In a large mixing bowl, combine the flour, coconut sugar, coconut oil, vanilla, baking soda, cinnamon, vinegar, and salt and stir well to combine. Add the chia seed mixture, which should have a thicker, gelatinous texture by now, and stir well. Add the shredded coconut and stir well again, making sure everything is uniformly distributed. Fold in the raisins.

3   Drop the batter by tablespoons onto the prepared baking sheet. Use wet hands or a fork to press the batter down into flat cookies, because they won't spread much while baking.

4   Bake for 10 to 12 minutes, until the edges look dry. (They might still be soft to the touch, and that's okay—they will firm up when cooled.) Allow the cookies to cool on the pan completely before serving. Store in an airtight container at room temperature for up to 5 days, in the refrigerator for up to 2 weeks, or in the freezer for up to 6 months.

NOTE: If you'd prefer a lower-fat cookie, you can replace ¼ cup of the coconut oil with ¼ cup mashed banana, and you can also replace the shredded coconut with rolled oats, if you'd like. The result will be softer and more cakelike, but still very delicious!

15-MINUTE PREP
KID-FRIENDLY
FREEZER-FRIENDLY

SPECIAL TREAT
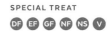

1 tablespoon ground chia seeds

3 tablespoons water

¾ cup gluten-free oat flour (see page 189)

½ cup coconut sugar

6 tablespoons coconut oil, melted

2 teaspoons vanilla extract

½ teaspoon baking soda

½ teaspoon ground cinnamon

1 teaspoon raw apple cider vinegar

¼ teaspoon fine sea salt

1 cup shredded unsweetened coconut

½ cup raisins

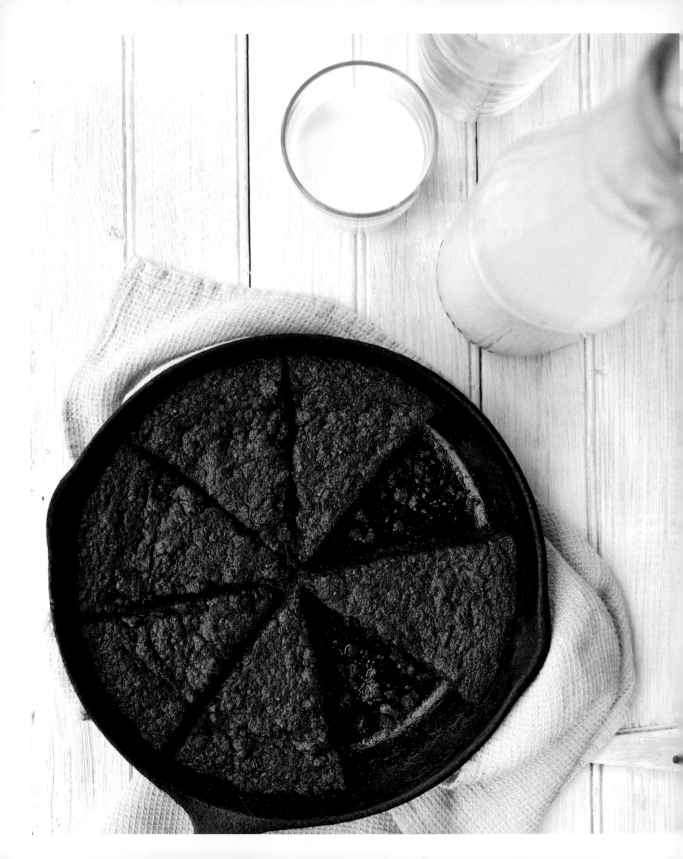

deep-dish chocolate chip cookie

SERVES 12 | $0.64 PER SLICE

15-MINUTE PREP
KID-FRIENDLY
FREEZER-FRIENDLY

If I were asked what my "last supper" would be, this deep-dish chocolate chip cookie would make the cut. It's warm and gooey right out of the oven and tastes unbelievably decadent when topped with a scoop of Creamy Vanilla Ice Cream (page 178). No one will believe this delight is made without white flour or sugar!

NUT/SEED/DRIED FRUIT

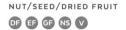

Coconut oil, for greasing

1 tablespoon ground chia seeds

3 tablespoons water

1 cup creamy cashew butter (see Note)

¾ cup coconut sugar

1 teaspoon vanilla extract

½ teaspoon baking soda

¼ teaspoon fine sea salt

¾ cup dark chocolate chips

1   Preheat the oven to 350°F and generously grease a 10-inch cast-iron skillet with coconut oil.

2   In a large bowl, combine the ground chia seeds and water and stir well to combine. Allow the mixture to sit for a few minutes to thicken.

3   At this point, stir any separated oil back into your store-bought cashew butter. Add the cashew butter, coconut sugar, vanilla, baking soda, and salt to the chia mixture and stir well to form a thick and sticky dough. Fold in the chocolate chips.

4   Transfer the cookie dough to the prepared skillet. Wet your hands with water (to prevent them from sticking to the dough) and press the dough evenly into the bottom of the skillet.

5   Bake for about 20 minutes, until lightly golden around the edges. Remove the pan from the oven and let the cookie rest for 30 minutes before slicing and serving. The hotter the cookie, the more soft and difficult it is to cut, although either way, it's delicious. Store leftovers in an airtight container in the refrigerator for up to 2 weeks or in the freezer for up to 6 months.

NOTE: For this recipe, I always use store-bought roasted cashew butter rather than my usual raw homemade version. Since this cookie is baked in a hot oven anyway, I think it's a waste of money to use expensive raw cashew butter, when the roasted variety is cheaper and more readily available. The store-bought option usually contains a bit of added oil and salt, so this recipe accounts for that. If you happen to find a brand with no added salt, increase the salt in this recipe to ½ teaspoon.

5-minute freezer fudge

MAKES ONE 9-INCH SQUARE PAN | $0.44 PER SERVING

NUT/SEED/DRIED FRUIT

(DF) (EF) (GF) (SF) (V)

1½ cups raw almond butter, at room temperature

¼ cup coconut oil, melted

½ cup raw cacao powder

½ cup maple syrup

½ teaspoon fine sea salt

2 teaspoons vanilla extract

This freezer fudge is my favorite healthy treat to keep on hand because it can be stirred together in just about 5 minutes and tastes like a decadent chocolate extravagance. Unlike traditional recipes, this fudge gets its texture from fiber-rich almond butter, which is loaded with protein and vitamin E, and it's sweetened with maple syrup, which contains calcium and iron. Paired with antioxidant-rich raw cacao powder, you'll be getting a boost of nutrition each time you satisfy your sweet tooth!

1   Line a 9-inch square pan with parchment paper and set aside.

2   In a large bowl, combine the almond butter, coconut oil, cacao powder, maple syrup, salt, and vanilla and stir until a uniform brownielike batter is created.

3   Pour the batter into the prepared pan and use a spatula to smooth the top evenly. Place the pan in the freezer to set until firm, about 1 hour.

4   Remove the pan from the freezer and slice the fudge into 1-inch squares. Store in an airtight container in the freezer for up to 6 months. This fudge will melt quickly at room temperature, so for best results, serve directly from the freezer.

NOTE: Do not be tempted to decrease the amount of coconut oil in this recipe, since it is key to the creamy, fudgelike consistency. You can decrease the measure of maple syrup for a darker chocolate flavor if you like.

no-bake brownie bites

MAKES ABOUT 12 PIECES | $0.66 PER SERVING

30-MINUTE RECIPE
KID-FRIENDLY
FREEZER-FRIENDLY

Although these bite-size treats are a simple combination of dates, walnuts, and cacao powder, they taste far richer and more decadent than you'd expect. Walnuts are a nutritional powerhouse, which have been shown to help reduce cholesterol as well as increase omega-3 fatty acids in red blood cells. Paired with mineral-rich dates, these brownie bites are a quick and truly guilt-free indulgence.

NUT/SEED/DRIED FRUIT

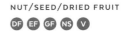

1 In a large food processor fitted with an "S" blade, grind the walnuts into a fine meal. Add the cacao powder, vanilla, salt, dates, and water and process again until a sticky, uniform dough is formed. (Be careful not to run the food processor too long, so that the walnuts don't get too hot and release excess oil into the mixture.)

2 Line a baking sheet or plate with parchment paper. Roll 1-tablespoon balls of dough between your hands and roll in additional cacao powder, then place on the prepared baking sheet. Place in the refrigerator or freezer to chill before serving. (When served directly from the freezer, the balls have a firmer texture than when stored in the refrigerator.) Store in an airtight container in the refrigerator for up to 2 weeks or in the freezer up to 6 months.

1½ cups raw walnut halves

¼ cup raw cacao powder, plus more for coating (optional)

1 teaspoon vanilla extract

¼ teaspoon fine sea salt

1 cup soft Medjool dates, pitted

1 tablespoon water

vegan chocolate cake

MAKES ONE 9-INCH CAKE | $0.63 PER SERVING

STARCH

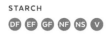

¼ cup coconut oil, melted, plus more for greasing the pan

1¼ cups gluten-free oat flour (see page 189)

1¼ cups coconut sugar

6 tablespoons cocoa powder

1 teaspoon baking soda

½ teaspoon fine sea salt

¾ cup water

2 teaspoons vanilla extract

2 teaspoons raw apple cider vinegar

1 recipe Chocolate Sweet Potato Buttercream (page 168; optional)

This cake has a surprisingly fluffy texture and rich chocolate flavor, just like the chocolate cake you grew up eating, but it's free of common allergens and is super-easy to prepare, calling for just one bowl and one type of gluten-free flour, instead of several gums and starches, which makes it slightly more temperamental. Be sure to let this cake cool completely before slicing, since it will be too soft and crumbly when warm. In addition to using parchment paper to line your pan, be sure to grease the top of the paper well to prevent any sticking. It's normal for a very thin film of cake crumbs to stick to the parchment paper when you remove it. Double this recipe if you'd like to make a two-layer cake (as pictured on the facing page).

1   Preheat the oven to 350°F and line a 9-inch cake pan with parchment paper. Grease the parchment paper with coconut oil.

2   In a large mixing bowl, combine the flour, coconut sugar, cocoa powder, baking soda, salt, water, vanilla, ¼ cup coconut oil, and vinegar. Whisk the batter together, ensuring that there are no clumps, and pour into the prepared pan.

3   Bake for about 30 minutes, until the top of the cake is firm to the touch. Allow to cool completely before cutting or frosting. Store in an airtight container at room temperature for up to 3 days, or in the freezer for up to 3 months, if unfrosted, or in the refrigerator for up to 1 week, if frosted.

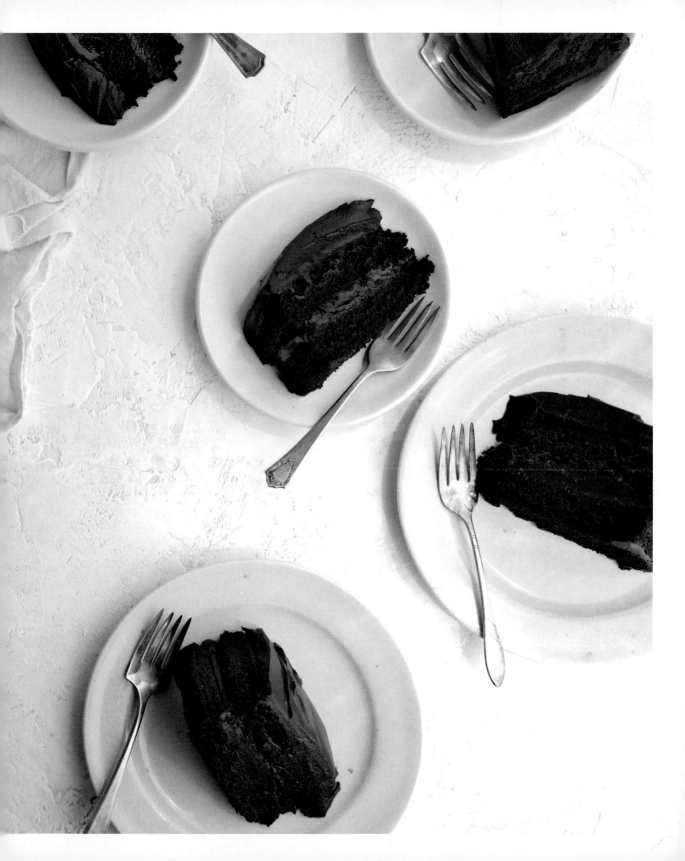

chocolate sweet potato buttercream

MAKES ABOUT 2 CUPS | $0.26 PER SERVING

STARCH

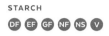

1 cup mashed sweet potato

6 tablespoons raw cacao powder, or more as needed

¾ cup maple syrup, or more as needed

¼ cup coconut oil, melted (see Note)

2 teaspoons vanilla extract

⅛ teaspoon fine sea salt

This buttercream is the perfect topping for Vegan Chocolate Cake (page 166). Most store-bought frostings are loaded with butter, shortening, and refined sugar, so this one is an upgrade, using fiber-rich sweet potatoes as the base and just enough coconut oil to give it a creamy and authentic texture. It's not as sickly sweet as the traditional variety, but it's still plenty sweet enough to make you feel as if you're eating a decadent chocolate cake. Unlike most naturally sweetened frostings, it can also be served at room temperature for a birthday party or special event. This recipe makes enough to frost a two-layer cake, but if you don't use it all, spread it into a lined pan and freeze it. It will firm up into a fudge!

1   In a high-speed blender, combine the sweet potato, cacao powder, maple syrup, coconut oil, vanilla, and salt and blend until smooth and creamy. (Feel free to add more cacao powder or maple syrup, to taste.) Place the frosting in the refrigerator to chill for up to 1 week until you're ready to use it—it will thicken as it gets colder.

NOTE: If you don't care for coconut oil, real butter can be used as an alternative—but then this recipe will no longer be dairy-free and vegan.

creamy cashew icing

MAKES ABOUT 1 CUP | $0.27 PER SERVING

15-MINUTE PREP
KID-FRIENDLY

This icing gets its creaminess from blended cashews, and when paired with a touch of honey, lemon juice, and salt, it tastes surprisingly similar to cream cheese frosting. (It probably won't fool anyone when eaten straight up with a spoon, but it's surprisingly authentic when served on Carrot Cake Cupcakes, page 171.) This is not the type of icing that can be piped or piled high on a cupcake, but a little bit goes a long way with this nutrient-dense alternative.

NUT/SEED/DRIED FRUIT

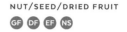

¾ cup raw cashews, soaked in water to cover for 2 hours

2 tablespoons coconut oil, melted

3 tablespoons raw honey

1 teaspoon vanilla extract

1 teaspoon freshly squeezed lemon juice

¼ teaspoon fine sea salt

2 to 4 tablespoons water, as needed

1   Drain the cashews and rinse well.

2   In a high-speed blender, combine the cashews, coconut oil, honey, vanilla, lemon juice, salt, and water—starting with just 2 tablespoons—and blend until completely smooth. Add another 1 to 2 tablespoons of the water if you need to help the blender break down the cashews—the mixture should be very smooth.

3   Chill the icing in the refrigerator for 2 hours before serving; this will help the flavors meld and the texture thicken a bit. (It still won't be a super-thick frosting.) Store in an airtight container in the refrigerator for up to 5 days.

NOTE: I recommend keeping your frosted baked goods in the refrigerator up until an hour before you want to serve them. Cakes and cupcakes will taste better at room temperature, since cold foods always have a muted flavor, but an hour should be plenty of time for them to come to room temperature without the icing melting too much. Alternatively, you can simply wait until right before serving to frost your baked goods to make sure the icing stays as thick as possible. Avoid letting frosted baked goods sit too long in a hot room—the icing will get runnier the longer it sits out.

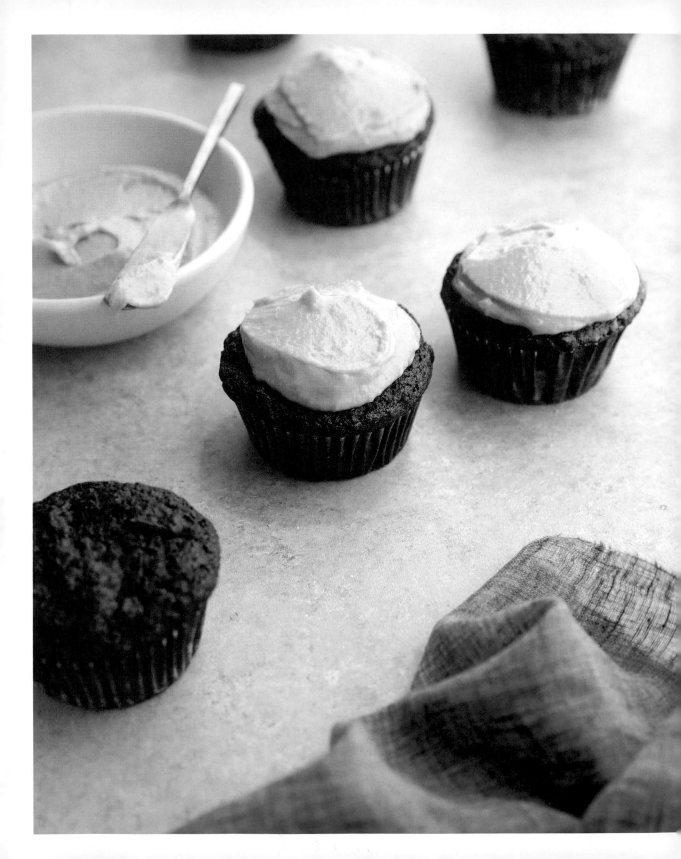

carrot cake cupcakes

MAKES 12 CUPCAKES | $0.42 PER CUPCAKE

Carrot cake has always been my preferred cake for birthdays and parties, so I'm thrilled to share a healthier version that is lower in sugar and higher in protein to help keep your blood sugar levels stable. These cupcakes are unbelievable moist and fluffy and hardly need frosting, but they also taste amazing with a dollop of Creamy Cashew Icing (page 169, as pictured here). If you need a nut-free frosting, try topping them with some Coconut Whipped Cream (page 184) instead.

SPECIAL TREAT

1   Preheat the oven to 350°F and line a standard muffin tin with 12 baking cups.

2   In a large bowl, whisk together the coconut flour, coconut sugar, coconut oil, eggs, cinnamon, ginger, salt, and baking soda until a smooth batter is formed.

3   Fold in the carrots, pineapple, and shredded coconut, then divide the batter among the prepared baking cups.

4   Bake for about 22 minutes, until the tops are firm to the touch. Allow to cool completely. Store leftovers in an airtight container in the refrigerator for up to 5 days. (They will start to dry out if left out at room temperature for more than 24 hours.)

NOTE: Be sure to use baking cups for this recipe rather than simply greasing the pan, because coconut flour is prone to sticking. I prefer to use silicone baking cups for guaranteed stick prevention.

½ cup coconut flour

1 cup coconut sugar

¼ cup coconut oil, melted

6 eggs, at room temperature

2 teaspoons ground cinnamon

½ teaspoon ground ginger

Pinch of fine sea salt

1 teaspoon baking soda

1½ cups shredded carrots

½ cup finely diced pineapple

½ cup shredded and unsweetened coconut (optional)

grain-free apple crisp

SERVES 6 | $1.18 PER SERVING

FILLING

2 pounds apples

1 tablespoon freshly squeezed lemon juice

¼ cup maple syrup

2 teaspoons ground cinnamon

½ teaspoon ground ginger

¼ teaspoon fine sea salt

TOPPING

1½ cups raw pecan pieces

½ cup shredded unsweetened coconut

1 tablespoon coconut oil, melted

2 tablespoons maple syrup

¼ teaspoon salt

¼ teaspoon almond extract

If you ask me, fruit crisps are better than pies because they are faster to prepare and have all of the flavor you love. This grain-free version is no exception, with a rich apple filling and buttery topping that you'll crave. I like to leave the peels on the apples, unlike traditional apple fillings, not only because it's much faster to skip the peeling process but also because the peel is where much of the nutrition lies. When baked, the peel becomes very soft and tender, just like the apples, and adds a great texture to the final dish. Serve with a scoop of Creamy Vanilla Ice Cream (page 178) on top for a truly decadent dessert!

1   Preheat the oven to 250°F.

2   To prepare the filling: Cut the apples into thin slices, about ⅛ inch thick, and place in a 3.5-quart Dutch oven. Add the lemon juice, maple syrup, cinnamon, ginger, and salt and stir to coat the apples well.

3   Place the pot over medium-high heat and bring the liquid to a boil. (You'll need to listen for the boiling, since the liquid won't cover the apples.) Once the liquid is bubbling, cover the pot and lower the heat so the apples can simmer for 8 to 10 minutes, until they are fork-tender.

4   To prepare the topping: While the apples are cooking, place the pecans and shredded coconut in a small food processor and process until crumbly. Add the coconut oil, maple syrup, salt, and almond extract and process again to combine.

5   Sprinkle the topping over the apples. Bake for about 30 minutes, until the top starts to look dry, then remove from the oven. Serve warm.

MAKE IT NUT-FREE: For the topping, combine ¾ cup oat flour, ¼ cup melted coconut oil, ⅓ cup coconut sugar, ½ cup shredded coconut, and ¼ teaspoon salt in a small food processor and process until crumbly. Sprinkle over the apple filling and bake at 350°F for 30 minutes, until lightly golden.

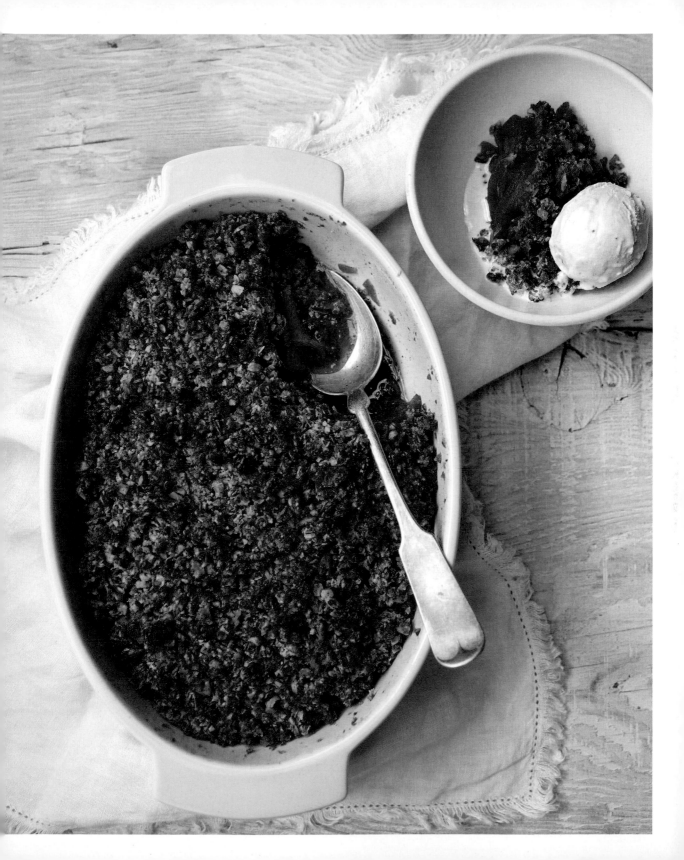

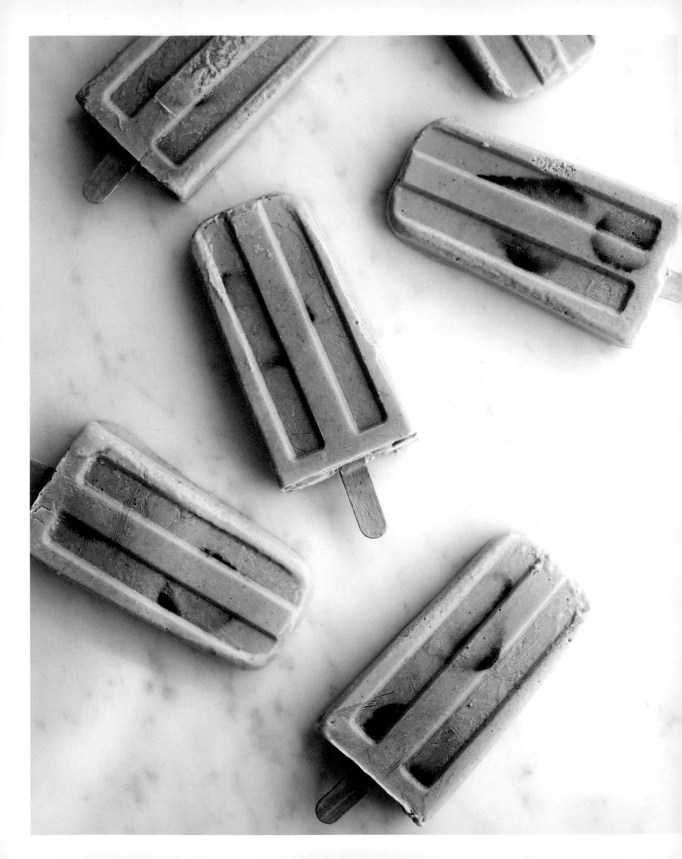

strawberries & cream freezer pops

MAKES 12 ICE POPS | $0.46 PER SERVING

15-MINUTE PREP
KID-FRIENDLY
FREEZER-FRIENDLY

These ice pops taste just like your childhood favorites but without the dairy or refined sugar found in the store-bought versions. I love to take advantage of fresh strawberries when they are at their peak of sweetness during the hot summer months, but you are welcome to use any fresh fruit you have to make a variety of seasonal and refreshing flavors.

SPECIAL TREAT

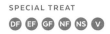

1 (15-ounce) can full-fat coconut milk

1 pound fresh strawberries, hulled

2 to 4 tablespoons maple syrup

1 teaspoon vanilla extract

1   In a blender, combine the coconut milk, strawberries, 2 tablespoons of the maple syrup, and the vanilla and blend until creamy. Taste and add the remaining 1 to 2 tablespoons maple syrup, if needed for sweetness. (Keep in mind that the ice pops will taste significantly less sweet once frozen, so the mixture needs to be slightly sweeter than you think necessary.)

2   Pour the blended mixture into 12 (3-ounce) ice-pop molds, leaving 1 inch of space at the top to allow for the frozen pops to expand. Insert wooden ice-pop sticks into each mold and place the molds in the freezer to set for 4 hours. Store in the freezer for up to 3 months and serve frozen.

NOTE: Feel free to add a few additional sliced strawberries to the mixture before freezing to create even prettier ice pops with small pockets of frozen strawberries throughout.

coconut lime pie

SERVES 12 | $0.64 PER SERVING

STARCH

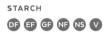

1 (15-ounce) can full-fat coconut milk, chilled overnight in the refrigerator

1 ripe Hass avocado, mashed

¼ cup coconut oil, melted

½ cup maple syrup

5 tablespoons freshly squeezed lime juice

1 Oat Flour Piecrust (page 185)

Coconut Whipped Cream (page 184) and lime zest, for topping (optional)

Many healthier desserts get their creamy texture from nuts, but this pie is allergy-friendly, using avocado and creamy coconut as its base. The avocado provides a beautiful green hue without the need for artificial food dyes, along with a hefty dose of vitamins K, C, and E; folate; and potassium. Paired with tart lime juice and naturally sweetened with maple syrup, this refreshing pie makes the perfect summer dessert.

1   Remove the can of coconut milk from the refrigerator, taking care not to shake it. Open the can and scoop out ½ cup of the thick layer of coconut cream from the top—you don't want any of the liquid on the bottom.

2   In a high-speed blender, combine the coconut cream, avocado, coconut oil, maple syrup, and lime juice and blend until completely smooth. Taste and adjust any flavors.

3   Pour the filling into the crust and place the pie in the refrigerator, covered, to chill until set, about 4 hours or up to 4 days. Slice and serve chilled, topping with Coconut Whipped Cream and lime zest.

NOTE: You can reserve the remaining coconut milk liquid for a smoothie the next day. If you'd prefer to avoid using canned coconut milk, add an extra ¼ cup coconut oil to the recipe in place of the coconut cream. The results aren't quite as light and creamy, but it still works.

Coconut and Nut Allergies
Although the FDA recognizes coconut as a tree nut, the American College of Allergy, Asthma & Immunology classifies coconut as a fruit, not a botanical nut, and has stated that most people who are allergic to tree nuts can safely eat coconut.[3] If you are allergic to tree nuts, be sure to talk to your allergist before adding coconut to your diet.

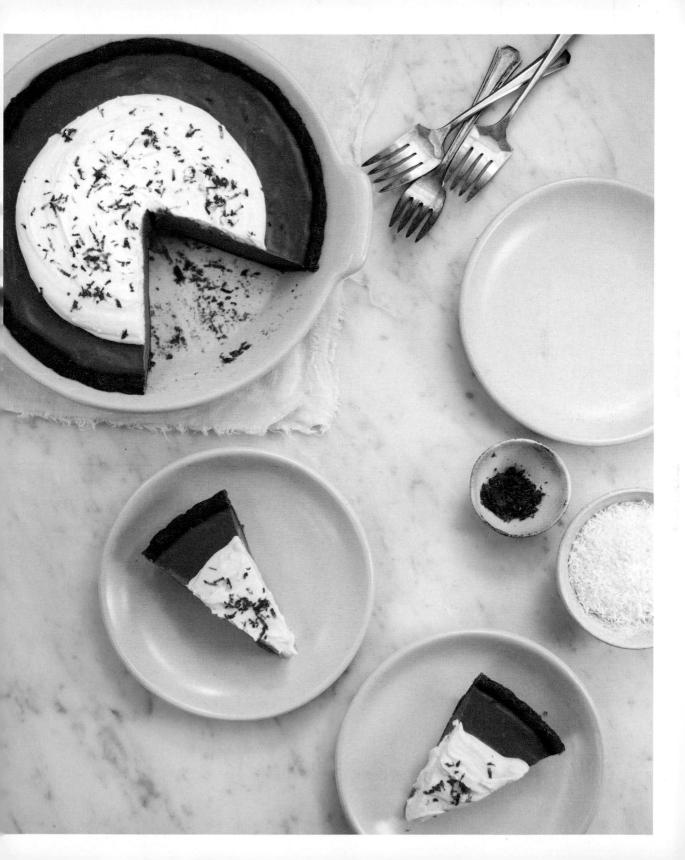

creamy vanilla ice cream

MAKES ABOUT 3½ CUPS | $0.76 PER SERVING

SPECIAL TREAT

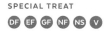

1 (15-ounce) can full-fat coconut milk, chilled

1 cup mashed sweet potato, cooled (see Note)

½ cup maple syrup

2 teaspoons vanilla extract

While my go-to ice cream is usually a quick blend of frozen bananas to create a fruit-based "soft serve," this coconut-based ice cream is much more decadent and authentic. Thanks to the use of an ice-cream maker, this dairy-free ice cream is churned into a consistency similar to the traditional kind made with heavy cream and sugar. Be sure to freeze your ice-cream maker bowl at least 24 hours in advance so it is fully frozen before getting started. Because this ice cream has no added thickeners or stabilizers, it will firm up when frozen, but you can thaw it on the counter for 30 minutes to make it scoopable again.

1   In a high-speed blender, combine the coconut milk, sweet potato, maple syrup, and vanilla and blend until completely smooth.

2   Pour the mixture into the chilled ice-cream maker bowl and process according to the manufacturer's instructions, about 30 minutes, until thick and creamy with a soft serve–like consistency. (The colder your ingredients are to start with, the faster they will thicken up.) Serve immediately. Store in an airtight container in the freezer for up to 2 months.

NOTE: I prefer to use white-fleshed sweet potato to keep this ice cream looking like vanilla ice cream, but it works just as well with the orange-fleshed variety, too. For potato baking tips, see page 14.

No Ice-Cream Maker?
Pour the ice cream into a shallow pan to freeze and then stir every 45 minutes until the desired consistency is achieved. It's more work than using an ice-cream maker, but it's still tasty.

instant hot fudge sauce

MAKES ABOUT ½ CUP | $0.33 PER SERVING

What I love about this hot fudge sauce is that it's loaded with fiber, has no added oil, and the taste can be adjusted easily as you go. Want a darker chocolate flavor? Add more cacao powder. Want it sweeter? Add a touch more maple syrup. If you need a nut-free alternative, swap out the almond butter for sunflower seed butter and adjust the sweetness to taste. Enjoy the instant gratification!

NUT/SEED/DRIED FRUIT

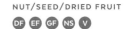

1   In a small bowl, combine the almond butter, cacao powder, maple syrup, 2 tablespoons of the water, and the salt and stir well to combine. Add the remaining 1 tablespoon water for a thinner consistency, if desired. Serve immediately. If you want the fudge sauce to be warmer, use a double boiler to gently heat to the desired temperature. Store leftovers in an airtight container in the refrigerator for up to 4 days.

2 tablespoons raw almond butter, at room temperature

2 tablespoons raw cacao powder

2 tablespoons maple syrup

2 to 3 tablespoons very hot water

Pinch of fine sea salt

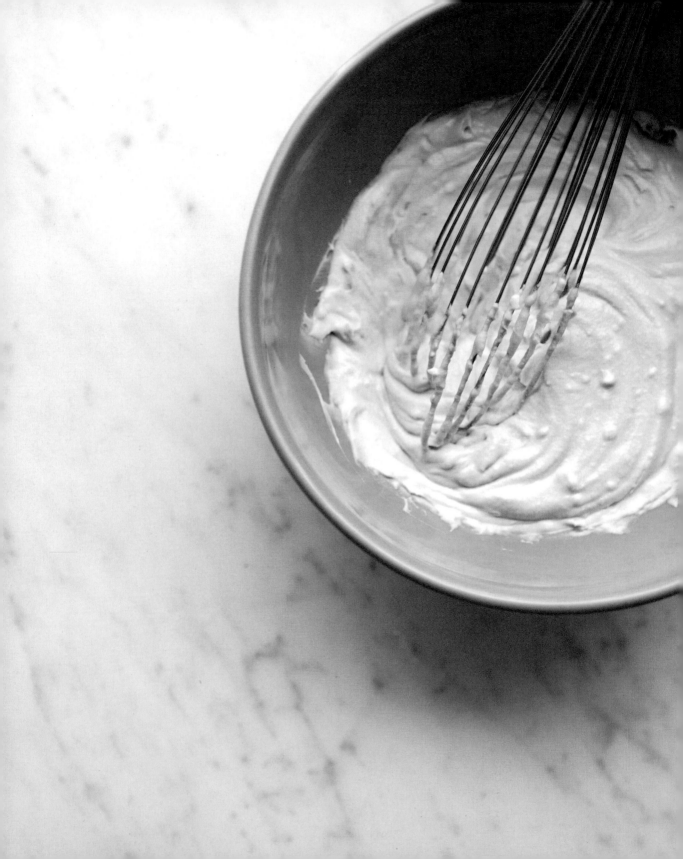

9 HEALTHIER HOMEMADE STAPLES

chocolate almond milk

MAKES ABOUT 4 CUPS | $1.71 PER SERVING

NEUTRAL

1 cup raw almonds, soaked for 1 hour and then drained (see box)

4 cups water

¼ cup raw cacao powder

2 teaspoons vanilla extract

8 soft Medjool dates, pitted

Chocolate milk was a staple in my family's refrigerator when I was a child, so this recipe is the perfect solution for those of us who still want to enjoy an occasional glass. It's made with a simple combination of almonds, dates, raw cacao powder, and vanilla for a rich, chocolatey drink that secretly packs some fiber and minerals, too.

1   In a high-speed blender, combine the almonds and water and blend until the almonds look pulverized and the liquid is creamy white.

2   Arrange a nut milk bag or fine-mesh sieve over a large bowl and pour the blended mixture into it to strain out the fine almond pulp. Squeeze well to extract all of the creamy almond milk and then rinse the blender container. (This plain almond milk can be used in any recipe calling for nondairy milk.)

3   Pour the strained almond milk back into the blender and add in the cacao powder, vanilla, and dates. Blend well until very smooth, then pour into an airtight container and chill for 2 hours before serving. Because this milk has no preservatives, it will last only 4 or 5 days in the fridge. (You can tell by taste when it goes bad.) Feel free to halve this recipe or freeze the extra for up to 3 months and thaw for later use.

NOTE: If you have difficulty locating or blending dates, you can replace them with ¼ cup maple syrup instead.

Don't Waste the Pulp

You can add the leftover almond pulp to a batch of Nut-Free Gingerbread Granola (page 38), although it won't be nut-free with that addition.

rice milk

MAKES ABOUT 3 CUPS | $0.11 PER SERVING

15-MINUTE PREP
KID-FRIENDLY
FREEZER-FRIENDLY

If you need a nut-free and nondairy milk, rice milk is an easy and super-affordable alternative. It is similar to making almond milk; you simply blend cooked rice with water and strain to create a light and creamy milk that is free of preservatives and fillers found in the store-bought varieties. I find that grain-based milks have a slightly starchy quality to them, making it seem as if they have a thickener added, and not surprisingly, they taste mildly of the grain that is used to make them. Enjoy this milk over your favorite cereal or, for a more satiating breakfast, try it with Nut-Free Gingerbread Granola (page 38).

NEUTRAL

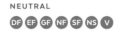

1 cup cooked rice of choice

3 cups water

1   In a high-speed blender, combine the rice and water and blend until completely smooth and creamy.

2   Arrange a nut milk bag or fine-mesh sieve over a large bowl and pour the blended mixture into it to strain out any remaining pulp. (There won't be a lot of pulp to strain out.)

3   Pour into an airtight container and chill for 2 hours before serving. Use or freeze the milk within 4 days for up to 3 months.

NOTE: This recipe can also be used to make oat milk, but I find that both rolled and steel-cut oats give the milk a slightly slimy texture that could be unappealing to some. To help minimize this effect, soak the oats in water for up to 4 hours ahead of time and then drain well.

TIME-SAVING TIP: This recipe comes together in minutes when you have prepared rice on hand. I like to make a large batch of rice over the weekend in my electric pressure cooker and then store the cooked rice in 1-cup portions in the freezer for quick weeknight meals and for use in recipes like this one.

coconut whipped cream

MAKES ABOUT 1 CUP | $0.13 PER SERVING

SPECIAL TREAT

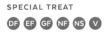

1 (15-ounce) can
full-fat coconut milk,
chilled overnight in the
refrigerator

1 tablespoon
maple syrup

½ teaspoon vanilla
extract

Coconut whipped cream is a fantastic alternative to the dairy-based variety, since it still whips up to a light and fluffy texture without using heavy cream or refined sugar. Be sure to use full-fat coconut milk, since it contains the most "coconut cream" needed for this dairy-free topping. This recipe works best using a can of chilled coconut milk, so be sure to place the can in the refrigerator overnight before you get started.

1   Remove the can of coconut milk from the refrigerator, taking care not to shake it. Open the can and scoop out the thick layer of coconut cream from the top—you don't want any of the liquid on the bottom, just the thick cream. (You can reserve the remaining liquid to make a smoothie the next day. The amount of cream can vary depending on each can, but the goal is to have about 1 cup for this recipe.)

2   In a large bowl, combine the coconut cream, maple syrup, and vanilla. Use an electric mixer to beat them together until the cream becomes light and fluffy, 2 to 3 minutes. Serve immediately. Store leftovers in an airtight container in the refrigerator for up to 3 days.

oat flour piecrust

MAKES ONE 9-INCH CRUST | $2.57 FOR THE WHOLE CRUST

This piecrust is an easy allergy-friendly alternative to traditional piecrusts. There's no need to roll it out with a rolling pin—just press the dough into a greased pie pan, making sure to press firmly into the crease of the pie plate so you get a crust that goes adequately up the sides of the dish and isn't too thick at the crease. This crust should work with a number of pies, particularly Coconut Lime Pie (page 176).

STARCH

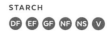

1 tablespoon ground chia seeds

3 to 4 tablespoons cold water, as needed

1 cup gluten-free oat flour (see page 189)

3 tablespoons coconut sugar

2 tablespoons coconut oil, melted

¼ teaspoon fine sea salt

1   Preheat the oven to 350°F and grease a 9-inch pie pan.

2   In a large mixing bowl, combine the ground chia seeds and 3 tablespoons of the water and whisk to mix. The mixture should thicken in just a few minutes. Add the flour, coconut sugar, coconut oil, and salt and stir well to combine. If the dough seems too dry to easily work with, add the remaining 1 tablespoon water.

3   Transfer the dough to the prepared pie pan and use your hands to spread it evenly into the bottom and up the sides, taking special care to make sure that the crease of the pan isn't too thick.

4   Bake for 15 minutes, then remove from the oven and allow to cool completely before filling. Store in the refrigerator for up to 1 week, or in the freezer for up to 3 months

pizza sauce

MAKES ABOUT 2 CUPS | $2.60 FOR THE WHOLE BATCH

NEUTRAL

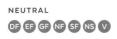

1 tablespoon coconut oil or extra-virgin olive oil

½ cup diced yellow onion

2 cloves garlic

1 (28-ounce) box or jar tomato puree (strained tomatoes)

½ teaspoon fine sea salt

½ teaspoon dried oregano

½ teaspoon dried basil

½ teaspoon balsamic vinegar (optional)

If you love marinara sauce, you're going to really love this pizza sauce. What sets pizza sauce apart is that the ingredients are simmered together longer, helping to remove the moisture that can leave a pizza crust soggy. This cooking process concentrates the flavor, making a delicious sauce that you can use in all sorts of dishes, such as Pizza Stir-Fry (page 151) or Cauliflower Baked Ziti (page 126).

1   In a large pot, melt the coconut oil over medium heat and sauté the onion until tender, about 10 minutes. Add the garlic and sauté until fragrant, about 1 minute more.

2   Add the tomatoes, salt, oregano, basil, and vinegar and bring the sauce to a boil. Lower the heat and simmer until the sauce has thickened, about 20 minutes. Taste and adjust any seasonings. Serve immediately. Store leftovers in an airtight container in the refrigerator for up to 4 days or freeze in individual portions for up to 3 months, so you always have pizza sauce on hand!

sunflower butter

MAKES ABOUT 16 OUNCES | $1.69 FOR THE WHOLE JAR

Sunflower butter is a fantastic alternative to nut-based butters for those with nut allergies. Store-bought varieties tend to include added oil, sugar, and salt because sunflower seeds are more bitter than other nuts, but I prefer to make it unsweetened and unsalted so that I can adjust the taste as needed on a case-by-case basis, depending on the recipe I'm using it for. I've also included optional additions here if you'd prefer to use it as a sandwich spread, similar to peanut butter. Be sure to try it in the Creamy "Peanut" Dressing (page 70).

NUT/SEED/DRIED FRUIT

(DF) (EF) (GF) (NF) (SF) (NS) (V)

3 cups hulled sunflower seeds

¼ cup coconut sugar (optional)

½ teaspoon fine sea salt (optional)

1   Preheat the oven to 250°F.

2   Spread the sunflower seeds in a thin layer on a large rimmed baking sheet. Warm them in the oven for 25 minutes to help them develop a nutty aroma and to blend more easily in the food processor.

3   Once the seeds are warm, pour them into a food processor fitted with an "S" blade and start processing them. Just like making any other nut butter, you'll need a bit of patience as they process, first turning into a finely ground meal, then forming a sticky ball, then finally turning into a creamy butter. The whole process should take about 15 minutes, but be sure to scrape the sides as necessary to keep the mixture moving.

4   Once the butter is smooth and creamy, feel free to add in the coconut sugar and/or salt and process again to mix well. Transfer the butter to a glass jar with an airtight lid. Store in the refrigerator for up to 2 months.

NOTE: If using sunflower butter in baking, it's important to know that sunflower seeds have a chemical reaction with baking soda and will turn your baked goods green. The result is not unsafe to eat, but it can be a bit shocking if you're not prepared for it. This reaction is something fun to keep in mind for St. Patrick's Day, when you might want a naturally green-colored baked good.

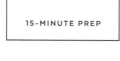

15-MINUTE PREP

fresh pico de gallo

MAKES ABOUT 2 CUPS | $1.00 PER SERVING

NEUTRAL

DF EF GF NF SF NS V

1 pound tomatoes, diced

½ cup diced red onion

½ cup diced green bell pepper

½ jalapeño chile, seeded and minced

1 clove garlic, minced

1 tablespoon freshly squeezed lime juice

¼ teaspoon ground cumin

¼ teaspoon fine sea salt

Store-bought salsa may often contain added sugar and preservatives, so this fresh pico de gallo is a quick and easy alternative. Simply stir it all together and serve. If you prefer a more blended, uniform dip, feel free to pulse it in a food processor until your perfect texture is achieved.

---

1   In a large bowl, combine the tomatoes, onion, bell pepper, jalapeño, garlic, lime juice, cumin, and salt and stir well to combine. (You may also process the ingredients together in a small food processor, if you'd prefer a smoother texture.) Taste and adjust any seasonings. Let the flavors meld for 15 minutes before serving. Store leftovers in an airtight container in the refrigerator for up to 4 days.

NOTE: Use this pico de gallo in my Cashew Queso (page 97) or Sweet Potato Queso (page 99) for a creamy and flavorful party dip.

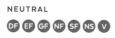

15-MINUTE PREP

guacamole

MAKES ABOUT 1½ CUPS | $1.00 PER SERVING

NEUTRAL

DF EF GF NF SF NS V

2 ripe Hass avocados

3 tablespoons freshly squeezed lemon juice

1 Roma tomato, chopped

½ cup finely diced red onion

1 clove garlic, minced

½ teaspoon salt

This classic dip is a staple in any healthy diet, and couldn't be easier to prepare. Use it for my Loaded Nacho Dip on page 108, or keep it on hand in your fridge for an easy snack!

---

1   In a large bowl, combine the avocados, lemon juice, tomato, onion, garlic, and salt and mash together with a fork. Taste and adjust any seasoning and serve immediately. Store leftovers in an airtight container in the refrigerator for up to 3 days. To help prevent browning, lightly press a piece of parchment paper to the surface and remove it right before serving again.

oat flour

MAKES ABOUT 3 CUPS | $0.50 PER SERVING

Oat flour is the easiest and most affordable type of gluten-free flour to make at home. Simply blend rolled oats in a blender or coffee grinder and you're done! Use this flour to make a number of crowd-pleasing recipes, such as Vegan Pumpkin Bread (page 46) or Vegan Chocolate Cake (page 166). Be sure to buy oats that are certified gluten-free if that is necessary for you, since many oats are processed in facilities that also process wheat and may risk cross-contamination.

STARCH

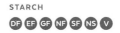

3 cups rolled oats

---

1   Pour the oats into a clean, dry, high-speed blender and blend until a fine flour is formed. Store in an airtight container at room temperature for up to 6 months.

NOTE: You can make a smaller batch of flour using a coffee grinder by blending only ½ cup oats at a time.

roasted red bell peppers

MAKES 2 ROASTED PEPPERS | $0.79 PER PEPPER

NEUTRAL

(DF) (EF) (GF) (NF) (SF) (NS) (V)

2 red bell peppers

Roasted red bell peppers are a flavorful addition to soups and sauces and are one of my favorite salad toppings. Sure, you can buy peppers in jars that come packed in oil, but it's even easier and more affordable to roast your own at home in just a matter of minutes. Simply prepare two or more roasted peppers over the weekend and save them for easy use in recipes or salads throughout the week.

1   Preheat the broiler.

2   Slice off the four squarelike sides of each pepper, discarding the stem and seeds in the center, and carefully removing the white pith with a knife.

3   Arrange the peppers cut-side down on a baking sheet, and place them directly under the broiler for 10 minutes, until the skins are blackened. (The more blackened the skins, the easier they will be to peel off later.)

4   Remove the peppers from the baking sheet and place them in a glass bowl with a tight lid, which will trap the steam they release. Allow the peppers to steam in the covered bowl for 20 minutes, or until they are cool enough to handle.

5   Using your fingers, easily peel away and discard the blackened skins, then save the roasted red peppers in an airtight container in the refrigerator for up to 1 week until ready to use.

NOTE: Use these peppers to make Roasted Zucchini Pesto Lasagna Stacks (page 133).

MEASUREMENT CONVERSION CHARTS

VOLUME

U.S.	IMPERIAL	METRIC
1 tablespoon	½ fl oz	15 ml
2 tablespoons	1 fl oz	30 ml
¼ cup	2 fl oz	60 ml
⅓ cup	3 fl oz	90 ml
½ cup	4 fl oz	120 ml
⅔ cup	5 fl oz (¼ pint)	150 ml
¾ cup	6 fl oz	180 ml
1 cup	8 fl oz (⅓ pint)	240 ml
1¼ cups	10 fl oz (½ pint)	300 ml
2 cups (1 pint)	16 fl oz (⅔ pint)	480 ml
2½ cups	20 fl oz (1 pint)	600 ml
1 quart	32 fl oz (1⅔ pints)	1 L

TEMPERATURE

FAHRENHEIT	CELSIUS/GAS MARK
250°F	120°C/gas mark ½
275°F	135°C/gas mark 1
300°F	150°C/gas mark 2
325°F	160°C/gas mark 3
350°F	180 or 175°C/gas mark 4
375°F	190°C/gas mark 5
400°F	200°C/gas mark 6
425°F	220°C/gas mark 7
450°F	230°C/gas mark 8
475°F	245°C/gas mark 9
500°F	260°C

LENGTH

U.S.	METRIC
¼ inch	6 mm
½ inch	1.25 cm
¾ inch	2 cm
1 inch	2.5 cm
6 inches (½ foot)	15 cm
12 inches (1 foot)	30 cm

WEIGHT

U.S./IMPERIAL	METRIC
½ oz	15 g
1 oz	30 g
2 oz	60 g
¼ lb	115 g
⅓ lb	150 g
½ lb	225 g
¾ lb	350 g
1 lb	450 g

RESOURCES

I rely on Amazon.com and other online retailers for ordering nonperishable goods easily and affordably. You can conveniently find all of my favorite pantry staples and kitchen tools here at detoxinista.com/resources. Or you can search for the following items at your local retailers.

INGREDIENTS

Almond Butter (Organic Raw)
Artisana
www.artisanafoods.com

Almonds (Organic Raw) and Almond Flour (Organic Blanched)
Nuts.com
www.nuts.com

Apple Cider Vinegar (Raw)
Bragg
www.bragg.com

Buckwheat Groats (Raw)
Bob's Red Mill
www.bobsredmill.com

Cacao Powder (Raw)
Navitas Naturals
www.navitasnaturals.com

Chocolate Chips (Allergy-Free, Dark)
Enjoy Life
www.enjoylifefoods.com

Coconut (Shredded Unsweetened) and Coconut Flour
Let's Do . . . Organic
www.edwardandsons.com

Coconut Aminos (Raw)
Coconut Secret
www.coconutsecret.com

Coconut Milk (BPA-Free)
Native Forest
www.edwardandsons.com

Coconut Oil (Extra-Virgin) and Coconut Sugar
Nutiva
www.nutiva.com

Coconut Water (Raw)
Exotic Superfoods
www.exoticsuperfoods.com

Harmless Harvest
www.harmlessharvest.com

Hemp Hearts
Manitoba Harvest
www.manitobaharvest.com

Honey (Raw)
YS Eco Bee Farms
www.vitacost.com

Maple Syrup (Grade B)
Coombs Family Farms
www.coombsfamilyfarms.com

Nutritional Yeast
Bragg
www.bragg.com

Oat Flour (Gluten-Free)
Bob's Red Mill
www.bobsredmill.com

Olive Oil (Extra-Virgin)
Bragg
www.bragg.com

Sea Salt (Fine)
Real Salt
www.realsalt.com

Sriracha
Sky Valley by Organicville
www.organicvillefoods.com

Tahini (Raw)
Living Tree Community Foods
www.livingtreecommunity.com

Tamari
San-J
www.san-j.com

———

TOOLS

Cast-Iron Cookware
Lodge
www.lodgemfg.com

Ceramic Bakeware
Emile Henry
www.emilehenry.com

Ceramic Knives
Kyocera
www.kyoceraadvancedceramics.com

Enameled Dutch Ovens
Le Creuset
www.lecreuset.com

Food Processors
KitchenAid
www.kitchenaid.com

High-Speed Blenders
Vitamix
www.vitamix.com

Mandoline Slicers
Benriner
www.amazon.com

Mini Food Choppers
Black & Decker
www.blackanddeckerappliances.com

Nut Milk Bags
The Raw Food World
www.therawfoodworld.com

Parchment Paper and Baking Cups
If You Care
www.ifyoucare.com

Pressure Cooker/Slow Cooker (Electric)
Instant Pot
www.instantpot.com

VitaClay
www.vitaclaychef.com

Silicone Baking Cups
Lekue
www.lekue.com

Spiralizers
Inspiralizer
www.inspiralized.com

Paderno
www.williams-sonoma.com

Waffle Iron
Old-Fashioned Cast-Iron

Rome Industries
www.romeindustries.com

Electric, Ceramic-Coated

Oster
www.oster.com

NUTRITION FACTS

While I don't recommend tracking your calorie or macronutrient intake or using those numbers to determine how "healthy" a recipe is, I realize that this information can be useful for certain medical conditions. Here, you'll find the total number of servings in each recipe, followed by the calories and macronutrients in each serving.

	SERVINGS	CALORIES	FAT	CARBOHYDRATE	FIBER	PROTEIN
2 SPEEDY SHAKES & MORNING FAVORITES						
Frosty Chocolate Shake	1	543	14 g	93 g	19 g	13 g
Sweet Tart Smoothie	1	466	2 g	113 g	15 g	4 g
Ginger Peach Detox Smoothie	1	358	1 g	89 g	10 g	5 g
Orange-Mango Creamsicle Smoothie	1	254	6 g	48 g	8 g	4 g
Frozen Chai Latte	1	473	16 g	80 g	10 g	9 g
Nut-Free Gingerbread Granola	4	409	32 g	25 g	4 g	14 g
Cream of Buckwheat Porridge	4	201	2 g	45 g	5 g	6 g
Morning Glory Snack Muffins	12	170	7 g	24 g	4 g	5 g
Cashew Butter Spice Muffins	12	195	12 g	19 g	1 g	4 g
Broccoli Cheese Egg Muffins	12	46	2 g	3 g	1 g	4 g
Mushroom & Leek Egg Bake	4	307	21 g	11 g	2 g	23 g
Vegan Pumpkin Bread	12	163	6 g	27 g	2 g	2 g
Freezer Oat Waffles	5	362	15 g	50 g	6 g	9 g
Skillet Breakfast Hash	2	212	10 g	4 g	2 g	14 g

	SERVINGS	CALORIES	FAT	CARBOHYDRATE	FIBER	PROTEIN
3 SALADS & DRESSINGS						
Knock-Off Italian Dressing	6	116	13 g	1 g	0 g	0 g
Balsamic Thyme Vinaigrette	8	137	14 g	4 g	0 g	0 g
Creamy Herb Dressing	8	94	8 g	4 g	1 g	3 g
Chopped Salad with Creamy Feta Dressing	4	242	16 g	17 g	7 g	10 g
Carrot Raisin Slaw	4	274	17 g	32 g	5 g	3 g
Chickpea & Avocado "Egg" Salad	2	223	10 g	27 g	7 g	3 g
Roasted Beet & Goat Cheese Salad	4	161	12 g	10 g	2 g	5 g
Pizza Salad	2	450	39 g	27 g	11 g	13 g
Creamy Kale Salad	4	310	15 g	39 g	7 g	10 g
Mediterranean Quinoa Salad	6	502	18 g	72 g	9 g	15 g
Summer Strawberry Spinach Salad	4	317	24 g	24 g	5 g	4 g
Crunchy Thai Salad with Creamy "Peanut" Dressing	4	367	28 g	29 g	5 g	7 g
Shredded Brussels Sprout Salad	2	242	18 g	14 g	5 g	8 g
Avocado Caesar Salad	2	103	7 g	7 g	1 g	4 g
4 SOUPS & SIDES						
Tuscan Bean Soup	4	279	4 g	53 g	15 g	4 g
Cauliflower & Leek Soup	4	87	4 g	11 g	5 g	4 g
Mock Mulligatawny Stew	4	262	8 g	44 g	6 g	3 g
Creamy Mushroom Soup	4	120	3 g	17 g	3 g	5 g
Mexican Quinoa Stew	4	315	4 g	56 g	10 g	12 g
Addictive Garlic-Roasted Broccoli	4	95	7 g	7 g	3 g	4 g
Creamy Cauliflower "Potato" Salad	4	236	9 g	35 g	6 g	6 g

	SERVINGS	CALORIES	FAT	CARBOHYDRATE	FIBER	PROTEIN
Soy-Ginger Green Beans	4	77	4 g	10 g	3 g	2 g
Cinnamon-Glazed Carrots	4	76	0 g	17 g	4 g	1 g
Slow-Cooker Cinnamon Applesauce	10	71	0 g	19 g	3 g	3 g
Quick Bread & Butter Pickles	20	15	0 g	3 g	0 g	0 g
5 GAME-DAY APPETIZERS & SNACKS ON THE GO						
Savory Sweet Potato Crackers	4	180	8 g	22 g	3 g	5 g
Cinnamon Oat Crackers	6	192	11 g	23 g	3 g	3 g
Cashew Queso	8	28	2 g	4 g	1 g	2 g
Sweet Potato Queso	8	43	0 g	9 g	1 g	2 g
Mini Pizza Bites	10	41	2 g	1 g	0 g	3 g
Easy Party Mix	6	200	18 g	8 g	3 g	5 g
Southwest Lettuce Wraps with Sweet Cilantro Dressing	4	185	7 g	26 g	11 g	8 g
White Bean & Rosemary Dip	8	88	3 g	12 g	2 g	4 g
Zucchini Hummus	6	88	7 g	6 g	2 g	3 g
Loaded Nacho Dip	8	179	6 g	31 g	9 g	9 g
Garden Spring Rolls with Creamy Tahini Dipping Sauce	4	390	27 g	36 g	4 g	6 g
Date Energy Bites	24	121	7 g	13 g	3 g	4 g
Nut-Free Chewy Granola Bars	12	130	3 g	24 g	2 g	3 g
Baked Parsnip Chips	2	77	5 g	9 g	2 g	1 g
Crispy Garlic Chickpeas	4	139	4 g	21 g	4 g	5 g

	SERVINGS	CALORIES	FAT	CARBOHYDRATE	FIBER	PROTEIN
6 COMFORT FOOD & CASSEROLES						
Sloppy Joe–Stuffed Sweet Potatoes	4	377	4 g	70 g	16 g	17 g
Spinach & Artichoke "Pasta" Bake	4	287	11 g	32 g	11 g	14 g
Philly Cheesesteak–Stuffed Spaghetti Squash	2	323	18 g	25 g	15 g	16 g
Butternut Mac 'n' Cheese	4	588	10 g	103 g	6 g	16 g
Overnight Quinoa Pizza	2	249	4 g	46 g	4 g	9 g
Cauliflower Baked Ziti	4	262	12 g	23 g	7 g	18 g
Roasted Vegetable Rice Bowls with Carrot Ginger Sauce	4	512	32 g	54 g	8 g	9 g
Speedy Black Bean Burgers	6	131	1 g	24 g	6 g	6 g
Roasted Zucchini Pesto Lasagna Stacks	4	239	17 g	17 g	6 g	9 g
Vegan Shepherd's Pie	4	395	5 g	73 g	15 g	18 g
Zucchini Bolognese	4	263	15 g	28 g	8 g	8 g
Enchilada-Stuffed Zucchini Boats	4	166	6 g	19 g	7 g	10 g
"Cheesy" Broccoli Quinoa Casserole	4	379	6 g	66 g	11 g	18 g
Comforting Vegetable Korma	2	649	43 g	63 g	10 g	12 g
7 SKILLETS & STIR-FRIES						
Butternut Stuffing	4	210	14 g	22 g	4 g	4 g
Rainbow Lo Mein	2	591	14 g	107 g	12 g	18 g
Zucchini "Pasta" Primavera	2	407	15 g	64 g	32 g	19 g
One-Pot Quinoa Fried Rice	4	388	8 g	63 g	8 g	16 g

	SERVINGS	CALORIES	FAT	CARBOHYDRATE	FIBER	PROTEIN
Pizza Stir-Fry	4	486	15 g	78 g	27 g	28 g
Singapore Sweet Potato Noodles	2	528	8 g	101 g	18 g	19 g
Pad See Ew	2	560	17 g	83 g	22 g	25 g
Cauliflower Jambalaya	4	171	5 g	33 g	12 g	10 g
Mushroom & Black Bean Tacos with Avocado Crema	8	64	1 g	11 g	4 g	2 g
8 SWEET TREATS						
Chewy Vegan Ginger Cookies	12	105	9 g	4 g	2 g	3 g
Coconut Oatmeal Raisin Cookies	16	102	6 g	12 g	1 g	1 g
Deep-Dish Chocolate Chip Cookie	12	202	12 g	21 g	1 g	3 g
5-Minute Freezer Fudge	25	128	10 g	8 g	3 g	4 g
No-Bake Brownie Bites	12	285	25 g	15 g	4 g	6 g
Vegan Chocolate Cake	10	207	7 g	36 g	3 g	3 g
Chocolate Sweet Potato Buttercream	2 tbsp	57	2 g	9 g	1 g	0 g
Creamy Cashew Icing	2 tbsp	116	8 g	10 g	0 g	2 g
Carrot Cake Cupcakes	12	172	8 g	23 g	3 g	4 g
Grain-Free Apple Crisp	6	413	28 g	40 g	7 g	4 g
Strawberries & Cream Freezer Pops	12	64	5 g	4 g	1 g	0 g
Coconut Lime Pie	12	158	12 g	12 g	2 g	2 g
Creamy Vanilla Ice Cream	7	191	10 g	24 g	1 g	1 g
Instant Hot Fudge Sauce	4	82	4 g	10 g	2 g	2 g

	SERVINGS	CALORIES	FAT	CARBOHYDRATE	FIBER	PROTEIN
9 HEALTHIER HOMEMADE STAPLES						
Chocolate Almond Milk	4	250	10 g	37 g	5 g	7 g
Rice Milk	3	12	0 g	3 g	0 g	0 g
Coconut Whipped Cream	16	42	4 g	1 g	0 g	0 g
Oat Flour Piecrust	12	99	4 g	15 g	2 g	2 g
Pizza Sauce	6	120	2 g	20 g	7 g	5 g
Sunflower Butter	16	158	14 g	5 g	2 g	6 g
Fresh Pico de Gallo	4	34	0 g	8 g	3 g	2 g
Guacamole	8	64	5 g	4 g	3 g	1 g
Oat Flour	½ cup	240	5 g	39 g	6 g	11 g
Roasted Red Bell Peppers	1 pepper	51	0 g	10 g	3 g	2 g

ENDNOTES

1: NO MORE EXCUSES

1. A. Pan, Q. Sun, A. M. Bernstein, M. B. Schulze, J. E. Manson, M. J. Stampfer, W. C. Willett, and F. B. Hu. "Red Meat Consumption and Mortality: Results from 2 Prospective Cohort Studies," *Archives of Internal Medicine* 172.7 (2012): 555. https://www.ncbi.nlm.nih.gov/pubmed/23497350.

2. Meggs, W.J. and Brewer, K.L., "Weight Gain Associated with Chronic Exposure to Chlorpyrifos in Rats," *Journal of Medical Toxicology* 3, no. 3 (2007): 89–93, 10.1007/BF03160916.

3. Barbara J. Rolls, E. A. Rowe, E. T. Rolls, Breda Kingston, Angela Megson, and Rachel Gunary, "Variety in a Meal Enhances Food Intake in Man," *Physiology & Behavior 26*, no. 2 (1981): 215–21, http://dx.doi.org/10.1016/0031-9384(81)90014-7.

2: SPEEDY SHAKES & MORNING FAVORITES

1. Juma M. Alkaabi, Bayan Al-Dabbagh, Shakeel Ahmad, Hussein F. Saadi, Salah Gariballa, and Mustafa Ghazali, "Glycemic Indices of Five Varieties of Dates in Healthy and Diabetic Subjects." *Nutrition Journal* 10, 1 (2011): 59.

2. O. Al-Kuran, L. Al-Mehaisen, H. Bawadi, S. Beitawi, and Z. Amarin, "The Effect of Late Pregnancy Consumption of Date Fruit on Labour and Delivery," *Journal of Obstetrics and Gynaecology* 31, 1 (2011): 29-31.

3. Susana Manzano and Gary Williamson, "Polyphenols and Phenolic Acids from Strawberry and Apple Decrease Glucose Uptake and Transport by Human Intestinal Caco-2 Cells," *Molecular Nutrition & Food Research* 54, 12 (2010): 1773-780.

4. B. J. Meyer, E. J. De Bruin, D. G. Du Plessis, M. Van Der Merwe, and A. C. Meyer, "Some Biochemical Effects of a Mainly Fruit Diet in Man," *South African Medical Journal* 45, 10 (1971): 253-61.

5. Allan S. Christensen, Lone Viggers, Kjeld Hasselström, and Søren Gregersen, "Effect of Fruit Restriction on Glycemic Control in Patients with Type 2 Diabetes—a Randomized Trial," *Nutrition Journal* 12, 1 (2013): 29. Web.

6. Magdalena Madero, Julio C. Arriaga, Diana Jalal, Christopher Rivard, Kim Mcfann, Oscar Pérez-Méndez, Armando Vázquez, Arturo Ruiz, Miguel A. Lanaspa, Carlos Roncal Jimenez, Richard J. Johnson, and Laura-Gabriela Sánchez Lozada, "The Effect of Two Energy-restricted Diets, a Low-fructose Diet versus a Moderate Natural Fructose Diet, on Weight Loss and Metabolic Syndrome Parameters: A Randomized Controlled Trial," *Metabolism* 60, 11 (2011): 1551-559.

7. Shirley Evans Lucas, Maureen Meister, Sandra Peterson, Penelope Perkins-Veazie, Stephen Clarke, Mark Payton, Brenda Smith, Maryam Mahmood, and Heba Eldoumi, "Mango Supplementation Improves Blood Glucose in Obese Individuals," *NMI Nutrition and Metabolic Insights* 7, (2014): 77.

8. "Survey Data on Acrylamide in Food: Individual Food Products," U.S. Food and Drug Administration. Accessed April 15, 2016. http://www.fda.gov/food/foodborneillnesscontaminants/chemicalcontaminants/ucm053549.htm

9. Tariq Ahmad Masoodi and Gowhar Shafi, "Analysis of Casein Alpha S1 & S2 Proteins from Different Mammalian Species," *Bioinformation* 4, no. 9 (2010): 430–35.

3: SALADS & DRESSINGS

1. Carol S. Johnston, "Vinegar: Medicinal Uses and Antiglycemic Effect," *General Medicine* 8, 2 (2006): 61.

2. Cynthia A.Thomson, Emily Ho, and Meghan B. Strom, "Chemopreventive Properties of 3,3-diindolylmethane in Breast Cancer: Evidence from Experimental and Human Studies," *Nutrition Reviews* 74, 7 (2016): 432–43.

5: GAME-DAY APPETIZERS & SNACKS ON THE GO

1. "Alpha-linolenic Acid," University of Maryland Medical Center. Accessed April 15, 2016. http://umm.edu/health/medical/altmed/supplement/alphalinolenic-acid

2. Yosra Allouche, Antonio Jiménez, José Juan Gaforio, Marino Uceda, and Gabriel Beltrán, "How Heating Affects Extra Virgin Olive Oil Quality Indexes and Chemical Composition," *Journal of Agricultural and Food Chemistry* 55, 23 (2007): 9646–654.

8: SWEET TREATS

1. S. Wang, C. Zhang, G. Yang, and Y. Yang, "Biological Properties of 6-gingerol: A Brief Review," *Natural Product Communications*, 9, 7 (2014): 1027–30.

2. Nafiseh Khandouzi, Farzad Shidfar, Asadollah Rajab, Tayebeh Rahideh, Payam Hosseini, and Mohsen Mir Taherif, "The Effects of Ginger on Fasting Blood Sugar, Hemoglobin A1c, Apolipoprotein B, Apolipoprotein A-I and Malondialdehyde in Type 2 Diabetic Patients," *Iranian Journal of Pharmaceutical Research* 14, 1 (2015): 131–40.

3. American College of Allergy, Asthma & Immunology (ACAAI), "Tree Nut Allergy," http://acaai.org/allergies/types/food-allergies/types-food-allergy/tree-nut-allergy.

ACKNOWLEDGMENTS

I am so grateful for all of the talented and caring individuals who have helped me bring this book to life.

To Julie Bennett and Steve Troha, thank you both for working with me again to bring this second book into the Ten Speed Press family. I am humbled to work with such an amazing team and appreciate the support from the whole crew at the Crown Publishing Group and Penguin Random House. Kaitlin Ketchum, thank you so much for masterfully editing my manuscript and helping me to make this book as user-friendly as possible. It has been such a pleasure to work with you!

I want to also thank my photographer Erin Scott for inviting us into her lovely home and for making these photos look so dreamy! These gorgeous shots wouldn't have been possible without the food styling talents of Ashley Marti, her assistants Allison Wu and Michelle Battista, along with the direction of Emma Campion and Ashely Lima. I also want to thank Rachel Perry for standing in when I couldn't be there, and Lizzie Allen for bringing this beautiful book design all together. What a dream team!

To my readers and fans, this book wouldn't be possible without your daily visits, comments, and emails. You all help keep my creativity flowing, and I am forever grateful for each and every one of you.

To my volunteer recipe testers, thank you for bravely trying my kitchen experiments, both good and bad, and for providing such honest and thoughtful feedback. These recipes are better because of you!

I couldn't have done it without the help of Karen and Kevin McNellis, Mike McNellis, Sue von Geyso, Courtney and Tucker Gilmore, Sara Maples, Kristina Saladino, Alex Henton, Jennie and Andrew Perry, Laurel Caes, Laura Sloofman, Alyssa Shrum, Susan Nee, Shannon Spezialy, Carrie Olson, Mary Kando, Chelsie Johnson, Brittany Tolman, Marcia Hoyt, Danae Littlejohn, Linda Ficke, Meghan Kelley, Mary Ellen Nye, Tina Cash, Chawna Dill, Rita Buhlmann, Pammy Josey, Elizabeth Santos, Karen Biebe, Lena Gonzalez, Kate Lunn, Kristy Bilbie-Bekius, Melinda Vita, Julia Silverthorn, Susan Peters, Heather Peters, Julia Bergin, Heather Miller, Jennifer Sage, Alison Moodie, Molly Campbell, Jennifer Gonzalez, Sabine Jentzsch, Kristin Kelly, and Julie La Bar. And a special thanks to my youngest taste testers, Charlotte, Finn, Max, Cora, Audrey, Beckett, and Penny.

To my parents, words can't thank you enough for your constant love and support. Not only are you the best parents a girl could ask for, but you make even better grandparents! Our little guy is lucky to have you, and I thank you for keeping him safe and entertained during this particularly busy time in my life. You really went above and beyond, and I appreciate it more than you know.

To my mother-in-law, Sue, thank you for always being around to help, giving Austin and me much-needed date-nights out, and for cleaning my kitchen every chance that you got. It certainly needed it!

To my son, I suppose I should thank you for turning into a picky toddler, as it has forced me to become even more creative when it comes to sneaking more nutrition into our family's meals and snacks. No matter what, you always manage to brighten my day and I cherish every minute that we get to spend together.

To my daughter, thanks for making *me* the picky eater this time around! It was no easy feat to develop these recipes while pregnant with food aversions, but I hope the result is a collection of recipes that truly everyone can enjoy—whether they are in the mood for healthful foods or not. We couldn't be happier that you have joined our family, and I'm so proud to have worked on this book with you.

Finally, to Austin, thank you for being the absolute best husband, father, and friend I could ask for. None of this would be possible without your support! Thank you for your patience as I made a mess of our kitchen each day, thank you for solo parenting when I needed the extra time, and thank you for all of the back rubs, late-night coffee runs, and taste testing some truly disastrous recipe ideas. I couldn't imagine my life without you!

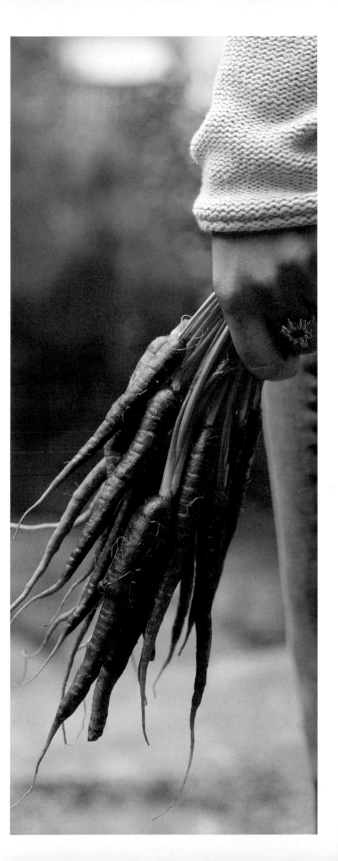

INDEX

Copyright © 2017 by Megan Gilmore
Photographs copyright © 2017 by Erin Scott

Published in the United States by Ten Speed Press,
an imprint of the Crown Publishing Group, a division
of Penguin Random House LLC, New York.
www.crownpublishing.com
www.tenspeed.com

Ten Speed Press and the Ten Speed Press colophon are
registered trademarks of Penguin Random House LLC.

Photograph on page 149 by Megan Gilmore.

Library of Congress Cataloging-in-Publication Data is on
file with the publisher.

Trade Paperback ISBN: 978-0-399-57902-8
eBook ISBN: 978-0-399-57-03-5

Printed in China

Design by Lizzie Allen

10 9 8 7 6 5 4 3 2 1

First Edition